Reducing the Risk
of Noncommunicable
Diseases

Reducing the Risk of Noncommunicable Diseases

Wesley P. Cushman, Ed.D.
Professor of Health Education
The Ohio State University

WM. C. BROWN COMPANY PUBLISHERS
Dubuque, Iowa

CONTEMPORARY TOPICS IN HEALTH SCIENCE SERIES

Consulting Editor
ROBERT KAPLAN
Ohio State University

Exercise, Rest and Relaxation— *Richard T. Mackey, Miami University*

Alcohol: Use, Nonuse and Abuse— *Charles R. Carroll, Ball State University*

Reducing the Risk of Non-Communicable Diseases— *Wesley P. Cushman, The Ohio State University*

Drug Abuse: Perspectives on Drugs— *Robert Kaplan, The Ohio State University*

Mental Health—*Henry Samuels, The Ohio State University*

Consumer Health—*Miriam L. Tuck, The City University of New York*

Venereal Disease— *Stephen J. Bender, San Diego State College*

The Human Body: Its Structure and Function—*Charles R. Schroeder, Memphis State University*

Environmental Health: A Paradox of Progress— *John Phillips, Jr., Sullivan County Community College*

Aspects of Sex Education— *Robert Kaplan, The Ohio State University*

Contraception— *Stephen J. Bender and Stanford Fellers, San Diego State College*

Communicable Diseases—*Deward K. Grissom, Southern Illinois University*

Copyright ©1970 by Wm. C. Brown Company Publishers

Library of Congress Catalog Card Number: 72—120074

ISBN 0—697—07331—9

Second Printing, 1971

Printed in the United States of America

Foreword

Health education is more than the primary phase of preventive medicine. Beyond the prevention of disease and the amelioration of health problems is its positive design to raise levels of well-being and liberate man's potential. Directly and indirectly it enables the individual to function most productively, creatively, and humanely.

One needs health to become educated and one needs education to develop and maintain health. Nor can one make full use of his education without it. Health is vital to the attainment of goals but we cannot preoccupy ourselves seeking it or in our obsession we shall fail to integrate all aspects of our development and performance. Health is a means to ends—the ends valued by the individual and society. Favorable modifications of health behaviors are essential to the attainment of these ends.

Contemporary Topics in Health Science offers a new and individualized format. Students and instructors can select and utilize those topics most relevant or most pertinent for the time available. Independent and class study, separately or concurrently, are enhanced by their organization. In this form they also provide greater opportunity to correlate health with other subjects.

Each book offers an up-to-date realistic discussion of currently significant health topics. Each explores its area in somewhat greater depth, with less trivia, than found in many textbook chapters. But they are designed to do more than merely present information. Within each are to be found more than partial explanations of facts. They are written by authors ranked by his professional peers as an authority in his field. They encourage the exploration of ideas, development of concepts, identifying value judgements, and selecting from a range of alternatives to enhance critical decision-making.

ROBERT KAPLAN, PH.D.
Consulting Editor

Preface

The health educator attempts to close the gap between scientific knowledge gained through research and clinical experience and the layman's knowledge and practice. Longitudinal population studies provide evidence that certain habits and ways of living can be instituted by young adults which will reduce substantially the chances of premature death, discomfort and disability from heart, stroke, cancer and diabetes.

In this booklet, a health educator discusses the specific steps important in reducing the risk of these diseases providing recent scientific evidence to support each measure. Factors in the control of other selected noncommunicable diseases of interest to students are presented. It is hoped that through the study of these materials the young person may better develop the concept that "how a man chooses to live effects his well being."

A glossary provides an adequate explanation of anatomical and physiological terms so the reader can gain an elementary understanding of the various disease processes.

The author is indebted to John C. Nash, Ph.D., Robert Kaplan, Ph.D. and George H. Bonnell, M.D. for their comments and suggestions.

Wesley P. Cushman

Contents

Introduction

A new descriptive term for an old concept in preventive medicine and hygiene is "risk reduction." Risk reduction programs propose certain behavioral patterns which substantially reduce a person's risk to disease. Longitudinal population studies provide increasing evidence that certain habits and modes of life increase the chances of premature development of specific noncommunicable diseases. The diseases have these characteristics in common: the cause is unknown, several variables are contributing factors in the development of the disease, the disease develops slowly over a period of years, early detection is important in control, and preventive measures can be taken now. Though the adoption of a risk reduction program does not guarantee that one will not develop the disease, it does increase his chances of adding productive years to his life and/or reduces disability and discomfort. Heart, stroke, diabetes, cancer, and other diseases in this group will be discussed. For those who have not had high school health or biology courses or who need to refresh their memories, an explanation of terms is included in the appendix.

CHAPTER 1

Cardiovascular Diseases

There are over 500,000 deaths from heart disease each year. It is most likely that this number will increase. On the positive side, this is good as it indicates that more and more people are reaching a "ripe old age." Unfortunately, about one-third of these deaths are among men in the prime of life; premature deaths that could be postponed for ten to twenty years. Women, for undetermined reasons, probably related to their sex hormones, have an advantage over men in respect to the risks of having heart attacks. It is not until after the age of sixty-five that the heart attack rate of women approaches that of men.

Scientists have learned that *coronary* heart attacks result from a condition in which the inner layer of the artery wall becomes thickened

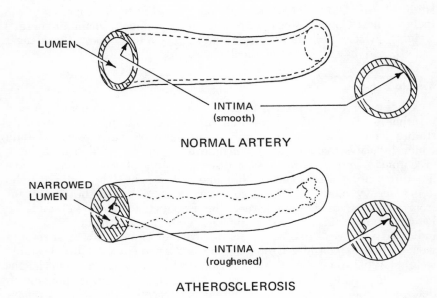

LUMEN

INTIMA
(smooth)

NORMAL ARTERY

NARROWED
LUMEN

INTIMA
(roughened)

ATHEROSCLEROSIS

1

and irregular by deposits of fatty substances. For reasons still not clear *cholesterol* and other fatty substances become embedded in the *intima* of the arteries reducing the size of the *lumen* of the blood vessels and roughening the artery lining. It is this process of *atherosclerosis* that sets the stage for heart attacks.

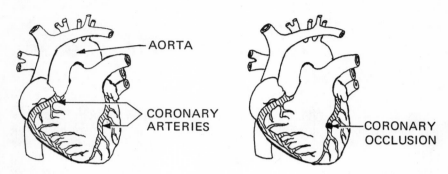

In their search for ways to prevent and control heart attacks and strokes, scientists have studied the living habits and medical records of thousands of people. For example, in Massachusetts, the Framingham Heart Study carried on by scientists of the National Heart Institute of the United States Public Health Service featured a painstaking search at regular intervals for clinical disease in over 5,000 men and women aged 30-62 at entry. (1) On the evidence of this and numerous other studies in the United States and abroad, risk reduction programs which include the following steps have been recommended: maintain normal weight, exercise regularly, don't smoke cigarettes, heed the danger signals, and have regular medical check-ups. (2)

Maintain Normal Weight

Obesity or excess fat tissue is considered to be the health hazard in atherosclerosis rather than what one weighs. Actuarial (statistical) studies from insurance companies over the years have provided data which indicates that overweight people have an increased risk of dying of coronary and *cerebrovascular* diseases. Most of these studies have not differentiated between obesity and overweight. The latter can be due to heavy bones and/or large amounts of muscle tissue as well as from an excess of *adipose* tissue. The Framingham study (1) and the Peoples Gas Company study by the Chicago Board of Health (3) indicated increased risk of coronary heart disease in obese men and women. One is considered obese if he is 20 percent over his desirable weight. What one should weigh cannot be determined from height and weight tables built on averages. The most scientific method to determine obesity is to measure the fat underneath the skin by a pinching method. This is not a practical method for the lay person to use. The adult in good health who has not been gaining or losing an appreciable amount of weight at the time can use what he weighed at 25 years of age as his standard. Perhaps the easiest method of determining if one is obese is to look in the mirror. (4) Stamler (5, p. 167) suggests using a yardstick placing it on the abdomen to learn if it touches both the sternum and the pelvic bone. If the abdomen protrudes, it will not touch both bones.

The physiological cause of obesity is a positive energy balance, but maintaining weight is more than reducing calories. One must follow three important guidelines: 1) maintain a balance between energy intake and output; 2) consume a nutritionally balanced *diet;* and 3) consume a diet that is psychologically satisfying.

Energy intake and output can be easily estimated. A person needs daily ten calories per pound of ideal weight to maintain his body metabolism at complete rest. Physical activity increases that need. The young adult leading an active college life increases his calory needs by about 100 percent. A day laborer, soldier, or athlete requires a 150 or 200 percent increase to maintain his best weight; whereas a sedentary person needs an increase of only 50 to 75 percent over his basal metabolism requirement. For example, Fred, a college man, of average build, six feet tall weighing 180 pounds will need: 10 (calories at B.M.) $\times$ 180 (pounds of ideal weight) = 1800 calories needed at rest; 1800 calories increased 100 percent for activity = 3600 calories needed daily. A pound of body fat represents 3500 stored calories. A person puts on weight in the form of fat tissue when for some reason, usually for healthy adults a change in the mode of life, his calory intake over a period of time rises above his daily needs. If this intake should be, let us say 100 calories a day he will gain between ten and eleven pounds a year. If a person is deficient in intake he will lose weight. For example, if a person wishes to lose a pound a week he must reduce his daily calory intake by 500.

Adults need a balanced diet to meet nutritional needs other than energy. To secure the appropriate amounts of protein, fats, carbohydrates, minerals and vitamins one needs only to choose daily servings from the basic four food groups:

1. Milk Group
   Children   — 3 to 4 cups.
   Adolescents — 4 or more cups (fortified with Vitamin D).
   Adults   — 2 or more cups.
   Provides needed calcium, also riboflavin, protein, and other essentials. Cheese and ice cream can replace part of milk.
2. Meat Group — 2 or more servings.
   Beef, veal, pork, lamb, poultry, fish, eggs, dry beans and peas.
   Provides needed protein, B vitamins, and iron.
   Liver once a week assures thiamine and iron.
3. Vegetable-Fruit Group — 4 or more servings.
   a. dark green or deep yellow.
   b. citrus fruit or tomatoes or raw cabbage.
   c. potatoes plus other fruits and vegetables.
   Provides: Vitamin C *mainly* through citrus fruits; also Vitamin A and minerals.

4. Bread-Cereal Group — 4 or more servings.
   Bread and cereals — whole grain or enriched.
   Provides: thiamine, protein, iron and niacin.

There continues to be controversy which components of diet are of paramount importance in atherosclerosis. Some scientists feel very strongly that *saturated* or animal fats are the villains. Certainly it is wise for those people who have too high a cholesterol count to replace saturated fats in their diet with polyunsaturated fats as much as possible. Diets for these people should be prescribed by a physician. Raising the proportion of polyunsaturates to saturated fats is accomplished by eating more fish and poultry in place of meat; using skimmed milk instead of whole milk; and in cooking, using vegetable oils instead of such solid fats as butter and lard. Cholesterol, a substance which our body manufactures, when taken in excess of what our body needs may be deposited in the arterial linings. Foods high in this substance are egg yolk, organ meats and shell fish.

Energy balance is probably more important than diet components. But if one begins to put on weight he can control it by cutting his calorie intake by reducing foods high in saturated fats and cholesterol.

Food Guide

Choose: fish, seafood, poultry, lean meats, salads, plain vegetables, fruits, cereals, plain breads, rolls, sherbert, angel food cake, gelatin.

Avoid: all fried foods, baked goods, creamed foods, high fat meats, stews, casserole dishes, pizza, cheese, butter, margarine, soups, sauces, salad dressings, ice cream, whipped cream (5, p. 175).

It is important in maintaining weight that one has a diet that is psychologically satisfying. "Crash" diets usually produce short term successes and long term failures because they do not offer the reducer any leads in regard to his long term need to reduce and to stay reduced. A weight program which provides for a small calorie deficit (not over 3500 calories per week) with foods selected from the basic four, and with a moderately increased program of exercise, has a much better chance of success. The person establishes a way of eating and exercising that is psychologically acceptable.

Obesity probably increases coronary heart disease risk by increasing blood levels of cholesterol and other *lipids,* increasing blood pressure, and increasing the work load of the heart. Maintaining one's normal weight reduces that risk.

Exercise Regularly

In the late forties and early fifties British investigators (6) obtained information on transport workers, postal workers, and civil service executives and clerks. Those more physically active such as conductors on double-deck buses and postmen were discovered to have less coronary heart disease than the less active workers such as bus drivers, clerks and executive officers. Since that time many studies made in Britain and the United States have shown that sedentary males are more susceptible to heart attacks than are physically active males. Levels of physical activity do not apparently affect the risk of coronary heart disease among females.

Scientists involved with the Framingham study found that the risk from heart attacks in men was sharply increased in those with sedentary living habits. "Least active" males had more than 3 times the risk of "most active" males. The risk of *angina pectoris* or coronary insufficiency in men was not appreciably affected by their habitual levels of physical activity. They report that in males sustained high levels of physical activity may confer protection against severe manifestations of coronary heart disease by stimulating the development of *collateral circulation* when the coronary blood flow is impaired by atherosclerosis. Also, that high levels of activity help to prevent overweight with the attendant benefits of lower fat levels, lower blood pressure and reduced cardiac work load.

It was mentioned earlier that an increase in exercise with reduction in calories was the most successful way to control weight. One study compared two groups of high school girls of similar age, height and grade. One group was obese, the other group of normal weight. Surprisingly it was found that the caloric intake of the obese group was lower than for the non-obese, but the obese girls were much less active. The researchers concluded that as a factor in obesity in this group of girls, inactivity was more significant than overeating. (7, pp. 37-44)

Another study learned that obese women walk only 1.9 miles a day compared to 4.7 miles for non-obese women; and that obese men walked 3.7 miles compared to 6.2 miles for men of normal weight. Until recently, nutritionists thought the only exercise needed was to "push yourself away from the table." They thought in terms of the amount of exercise it takes to burn a pound of fat such as walking thirty miles. What was overlooked was the point that one does not have to walk the 30 miles in a day. If one walks 3 miles a day, he thus accounts for a pound of weight in 10 days or 36.5 pounds in a year. (8, pp. 33, 80)

In adults big gains in weight are almost always preceded by a period of inactivity caused by an injury or an environmental change such as moving from active work to a desk job. It is helpful to watch one's weight by "weighing in" once a week in the early morning before breakfast and after urination. If one finds that he is more than 10 percent above what he should weigh, he should reduce to his best weight slowly. As previously mentioned combining moderate exercise with a reduction in calories is the easiest and more comfortable way to provide the energy deficit needed.

Exercise programs should be selected by the individual depending on his physical condition. If one has not exercised for some time he should start lightly and work up gradually to a vigorous program that

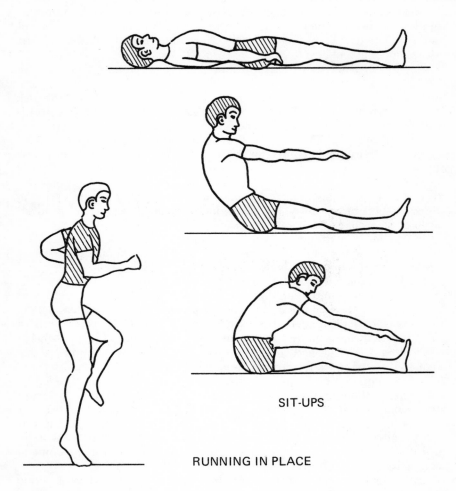

SIT-UPS

RUNNING IN PLACE

is best for him. The college student will gain most by participating in a sports program but those people who are short on time and facilities will find a simple routine consisting of four exercises carried on for ten minutes a day, three, preferably four times per week is all that is necessary.

The four exercises: running, sit-ups, push-ups and flutter kicks provide a minimum of total body development. Significant results can be gained for one can gradually increase the intensity without prolonging the time.

Running in place develops cardiovascular endurance. The person runs ten seconds, rests ten seconds, runs again. He takes it easy at first and then builds up to his full speed for the ten second intervals. Ten runs are sufficient. If room permits he can jog (run, walk, run) instead of running in place. This puts less strain on the bones and joints of the legs.

Sit-ups strengthen the abdominal muscles. Weak abdominal muscles are often a predisposing factor in low back pain and a front paunch. Sit-ups should be done on a two-count over a two minute period working up to forty. For middle age people 20 is sufficient.

Push-ups develop strength in the shoulders and arms. They should be done in a two-count. Fifteen to twenty push-ups is a reasonable goal. Older people and girls who may have difficulty with this exercise can modify it by having the knees touch the floor rather than a straight back and legs with toes on the floor. Intensity can be increased as one gains strength.

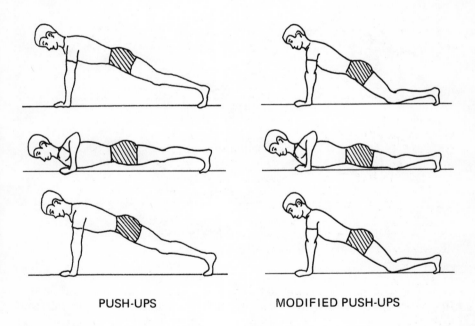

PUSH-UPS   MODIFIED PUSH-UPS

Flutter kicks are performed as in the Australian crawl in swimming. Head and chest off the floor, arms to side then alternate leg kicks with leg straight but relaxed. Forty kicks are sufficient.

For persons over thirty, programs involving jogging, sit-ups, and others should not be begun until after a medical evaluation.

Excellent inexpensive pamphlets on exercises suited to one's condition and age are available. (9, 10)

Dr. Jeremiah Stamler in *Your Heart Has Nine Lives,* (11, p. 115) discusses several studies which show that exercise may also be an important factor in lowering blood cholesterol levels. He is quick to point out, however, that the interplay of diet and exercise is complex and we cannot as yet conclude that exercise alone lowers the levels. Also, that the significant differences in rates of heart disease are between light workers and heavy workers.

Though the evidence is not completely in, we may say regular moderate exercise is important to the risk reduction program because of its possible influences on fat metabolism, collateral circulation, *coagulation* mechanism and its importance in weight control.

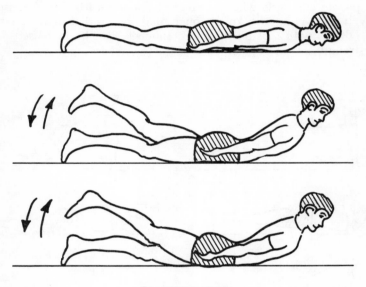

FLUTTER KICK

Don't Smoke Cigarettes

The acute cardiovascular effects of smoking on man are primarily the results of nicotine contained in tobacco smoke. After one or two cigarettes most persons will show an increase in resting heart rate of 15-25 beats per minute, a rise in blood pressure of 10-20 millimeters and an increase in cardiac output. A *vasoconstriction* of the blood vessels in the fingers and toes takes place while smoking with a consequent drop in blood flow and temperature. The Surgeon General's report on *Smoking and Health* concludes, however, that these acute effects do not account well for the observed association between smoking and coronary heart disease (12, p. 320). The report does cite, however, study after study establishing that male cigarette smokers have a higher death rate from coronary disease than non-smoking males.

The Framingham study shows that cigarette smoking increases the risk of severe manifestations of coronary heart disease. The risk of "heart attacks" among heavy cigarette smokers was about twice that of non-smokers. Low risk among pipe and cigar smokers suggests that tobacco smoke must be inhaled to produce its harmful effects. When a smoker gives up the habit, his risk quickly reverts to the low risk level of those who have never smoked. A marked increase of sudden deaths occurred among cigarette smokers and the risk of sudden death increased with the number of cigarettes smoked. The risk of sudden death among heavy cigarette smokers may be as high as five times that of non-smokers. Cigarette smoking was not related to angina pectoris nor was the duration of the cigarette smoking habit related to coronary heart disease risk. (13)

The Surgeon General's review of studies on smoking and coronary heart disease concludes that there is a significant association between cigarette smoking and the incidence of *myocardial infarction* and sudden death in males, especially in middle life. Angina pectoris, which indicates advanced coronary atherosclerosis is less closely associated with smoking than is myocardial infarction, and this suggests that any causal role of smoking in heart disease should relate more to acute occlusive mechanisms such as intravascular *thrombosis* or coronary spasm, than to the development of chronic arterial disease (12, p. 325).

The Framingham investigators concluded on the basis of the evidence they collected on the relationship of cigarette smoking and heart disease that it pays to quit now. (13) How do you quit?

Quitting smoking is not as easy as one thinks as any veteran smoker who has tried it can tell you. Tomkins (14) developed a model for smoking that relates smoking behavior to the sucking response which in infancy relieves discomfort or distress and promotes such positive affects as enjoyment and satisfaction. The basis for smoking may be the innate affect of the sucking response but the smoker may have learned to use smoking to make him less afraid, less disgusted or to give him a lift of excitement. If he has ceased to use smoking to reduce distress or to get a lift, we label him as a "habitual" smoker. He is hardly aware that he is smoking. A "positive" smoker is one who experiences excitement or finds a cigarette relaxing. The "negative" smokers use smoking to reduce tensions and distress. The "addicted" smokers smoke for any reason, for positive and negative affects. Knowing how one smokes may be useful in helping one to quit. For example, the habitual smoker usually has little trouble stopping as his smoking is not related to specific psychological conditions. If he carries his cigarettes in his shirt pocket, he can cut the pockets off so he must carry them elsewhere. He then becomes conscious of how often he is reaching for a cigarette. This may be all the help he needs.

Daniel Horn (15) has developed a model for smoking behavior change which shows the complexity of smoking. No one should feel guilty because he does not have the so called "will power" to quit smoking. For some people mastery of their own lives, that is, the ability to exert self-control is a strong enough motive but others may be motivated by the health risks or the exemplar role (setting an example for their children) or economics or several of these or none. Many will need an alternative psychological mechanism to substitute for smoking. Environmental forces make it difficult to quit: mass media promote it, friends and family continue to smoke, and, at present at least, smoking is still a most acceptable form of behavior. As such situations change it may become easier for one to stop.

It is estimated that over two-thirds of adult smokers have tried to stop with over thirty percent of these being off for over a year. So a smoker can quit and here are some of the ways that people have found to be helpful (16):

1) Think of stopping not as self-denial but as self-betterment.
2) Set a date to quit.
   Cut down gradually. Smoke only once an hour then every other hour and so on.
   Carry your cigarettes in another pocket.
   Shift to a brand you don't like.
   Find out under what situations you smoke.
3) Become well informed on the risks of smoking.
   Each night after going to bed review the facts you know about the risks of cigarette smoking.
After you quit and you are tempted to light up, try these:
Drink water.
Chew sugarless gum.
Breathe deeply.
Use an inhaler.
After meals use a mouth wash.
Ride in "no smoking" cars when commuting.
Avoid coffee breaks, if others smoke.
Exercise if you become irritable.
Change your evening habits, if you tend to smoke heavily at this time,
   e.g., read a book instead of watching T.V., take the dog out for a walk.

Remember you'll add an average of 6 1/2 years to your retirement pleasures and enjoy the taste of food and the smell of fresh air once again.

Heed the Danger Signals

Angina pectoris may develop after a person has had one or more heart attacks or may appear before a serious attack occurs. The pain occurs beneath the breast bone and may give the person a feeling of tightness or sense of constriction. It may radiate from the chest to shoulders and down the arm. It is a sign that the heart is not getting enough oxygen. It may be brought on by exercise and strong emotion. Chest discomfort can come from other causes including indigestion but in middle-aged and older people such discomfort should be reported to a physician.

Have Periodic Medical Check-ups

The annual medical check-up may catch cardiovascular disease at a time when much can be done to control or prevent further damage. Certain risk factors such as high blood pressure and high cholesterol levels and a tendency toward diabetes can be discovered only through a medical examination. The risk from these conditions can often be reduced through changes in habits and medication.

Many people between the age of 35-50 are unaware that they have high blood pressure which is a major risk factor for premature athero-sclerotic disease, a fact which has been documented in numerous studies (3, p. 236). Essential *hypertension* is a persistently high blood pressure exceeding 90 millimeters of mercury when the heart is at rest (*diastolic* pressure). It may pass through a transitional stage when the blood pressure rises only occasionally, then more frequently and finally re-mains at a higher level. Unfortunately, it seldom produces symptoms which are recognized by the person who has it. The physician can detect elevated blood pressure with an instrument called a *sphygmo-manometer*, an instrument using a rubber cuff and mercury columns which is familiar to most everybody. He will want to repeat measure-ments if he discovers an elevated pressure because blood pressure often goes up temporarily when a person is nervous. The doctor will also inspect the blood vessels in the *retina* of the eye. These can be seen through the pupil and lens by use of a small bright light. Retinal blood vessels often show the damage done by hypertension so the physician can judge the severity of the disease. If hypertension is present further tests are indicated such as an *electrocardiogram* (EKG) and chest X-ray to determine if the heart has been affected. Certain kidney tests may be performed to rule out that small percent of hypertension that may be due to other causes. The death rate from hypertension can be dra-matically reduced by diet and drug treatment.

Higher than normal cholesterol levels can only be determined by a physician. Middle-aged persons with *hypercholesterolemia* experience three or four times as many heart attacks as those with low normal serum levels. The Framingham study concluded that normal should be less than 215 milligrams percent and a reading above 250 would be high. Cholesterol levels as discussed previously can be reduced by diet and exercise which in these cases should be prescribed by the physician.

Diabetes mellitus is a major factor in atherosclerotic disease. It will be discussed later but is mentioned here as it can be tested for by the physician during the annual medical examination.

Treatment for Coronary Heart Disease

Over seventy-five percent of people survive their initial sudden, acute heart attack and eighty percent of those return to work. It is most important that the patient realize he can recover and will not be a burden. Emotional support from his family and friends as well as his doctor is basic to all other treatment.

Immediately following his attack the patient must have complete rest. In the hospital he will receive drugs to relieve his pain, to keep him quiet, and to lessen his anxiety. He will be given oxygen so the heart does not have to work as hard. He will be kept in the hospital for a period of time where medicines to restore falling blood pressure, to stimulate the heart, and to promote good rhythm, and where a defibrillator to straighten out heart muscle twitching, and an electro-cardiogram to check on the efficiency of the heart will be available. The doctor may give him anticoagulants to prevent thrombi and emboli forming.

Eventually the patient will sit up, begin caring for himself, and then start walking. His damaged heart tissue will have healed and collateral circulation will have been established. When he goes home, he'll have to adopt the habits recommended in the risk reduction program: appropriate eating, no smoking, moderate exercise, and periodic check-ups. He'll probably be back at his old job and playing better golf than he ever did because he spreads his 36 holes over the week rather than concentrates them into Saturday and Sunday. He may have to ease up as emotional stress, particularly over a period of time, may bring on a heart attack if arteries have become sclerotic. The chances are good that he'll enjoy life better than he did before his attack.

Strokes

During the fourteen years surveillance of the population in the Framingham study (17) 133 documented cases of *stroke* occurred. A detailed analysis showed clear cut differences between those who suffered strokes and those who did not. Atherosclerotic brain *infarction*, that is, brain damage due to blockage of the cerebral blood vessels, accounted for more than sixty percent of the strokes. Like coronary heart disease this disease increases with age but unlike coronary heart disease which develops some twenty years earlier in men than in women, *cerebrovascular* disease strikes without regard to sex. Hypertension seems to be a most serious risk factor in developing stroke. Most people with normal blood pressure do not suffer from strokes. People with elevated cholesterol levels have an increased risk of stroke and when hypertension and a high cholesterol level are both present the risk increases. As one might suspect, diabetics, particularly if high blood pressure is present, have an increased risk. Obesity only moderately increases a person's risk of a cerebrovascular accident.

What does all this mean to the young adult? It means that the risk reduction program recommended for coronary heart disease is equally sound for preventing atherosclerotic brain infarction. Maintain appropriate weight, exercise moderately, have regular medical check-ups, and heed the danger signals which are in the case of stroke: headaches, difficulties in vision, dizziness, fainting spells, numbness of hand or

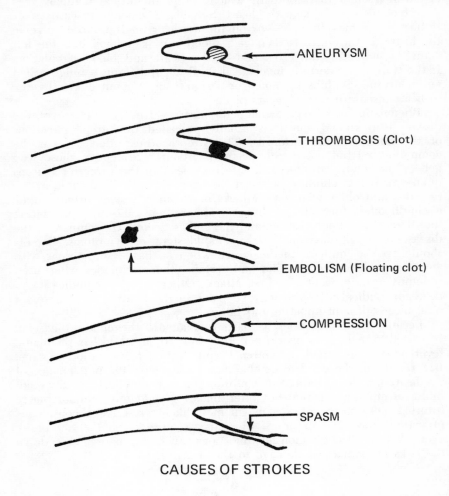

ANEURYSM

THROMBOSIS (Clot)

EMBOLISM (Floating clot)

COMPRESSION

SPASM

CAUSES OF STROKES

face, paralysis, difficulty in speaking, poor memory, and personality changes (18).

The other major type of stroke results when an artery breaks and there is intracranial bleeding. Arteries may be weakened from defects before birth, infections, as well as by atherosclerosis and high blood pressure. The strokes among young people are usually due to a *congenital* defect known as an *aneurysm* or an *embolus* formed in a heart damaged by rheumatic fever. Good medical care reduces the risk of stroke from these causes.

Infections Causing Heart Disease

The risk reduction program recommended above relates to heart attacks and strokes resulting from atherosclerosis. There are other forms of cardiovascular diseases with which adults should be familiar.

Infections can damage the heart. Syphilis, a venereal disease, in its tertiary stage may form *lesions* on the *aorta* or on the aortic valve in the heart. If the valve is damaged, blood can seep back into the left ventricle impairing the efficiency of the heart and blood circulation. If the wall of the aorta is involved it weakens and forms a bulge called an aneurysm. Syphilis accounts for a significant percent of deaths due to heart disease before 50 years of age.

Rheumatic fever may damage the heart valves. The cause of the disease is unknown, but it is usually preceded by "strep" infections of the nose, throat, or tonsils. The streptococcus infections can be communicated but not rheumatic fever. About 3 percent of those who get "A" hemolytic streptococcal infection develop the fever for reasons unknown. It hits children between the ages of 5 and 15. People in the twenties and older who have attacks of rheumatic fever usually show a childhood history of the disease. The responsibility for preventing the disease falls upon parents and the child's doctor. Unfortunately, the disease does not have any early reliable signs or symptoms. Parents should take a child for medical care when he has a sore throat with any degree of fever. Penicillin and certain other antibiotics when used promptly, can prevent the first attack. Other symptoms indicating a need for medical attention may be pains in the joints, pallor, frequent nose bleeds, loss of appetite and fatigue.

Because rheumatic fever is hard to diagnose the child's physician will need to make tests over a period of time. If the child has rheumatic fever he will need bed rest, often hospitalization for a period of time. Bed rest helps the child to combat the disease with the best chance of the heart not being damaged. Unfortunately, rheumatic fever does not build an immune reaction but often makes a child more vulnerable to future attacks so the physician will most likely prescribe a continuous preventive medicine program. This may require *chemotherapy* orally every day or through monthly injections. Such a program cuts down the risks of permanent damage to the heart (19).

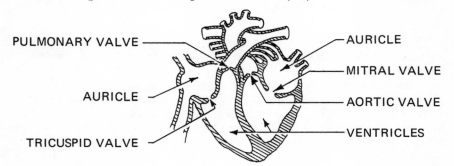

PULMONARY VALVE ——————— AURICLE

——— MITRAL VALVE

AURICLE ———— AORTIC VALVE

——— VENTRICLES

TRICUSPID VALVE ———

Inborn Heart Disease

Some people are born with heart or circulatory defects which we refer to as *congenital*. These defects exist because the heart or a major blood vessel near the heart has failed to develop normally. These defects are of many types and may occur singly or in combination. Fortunately, such conditions seriously affect less than one percent of all babies.

Seventy-five percent of all the common inborn heart defects can be corrected or corrected in part by surgical procedures. *Patent ductus* is a passageway in the newborn infant which connects the pulmonary artery and the aorta. It exists in the fetus because the blood does not circulate to the lungs for its oxygen. If it does not close soon after birth it allows blood that should be circulating through the body to pass back and forth between the heart and the lungs. Circulation of the blood of the child may be lessened if the *septum* (the muscle wall) between either the *auricles* or *ventricles* does not close off properly thereby leaving a hole. *Coarctation* or narrowing the aorta reduces the ability of this the biggest of blood vessels to transport blood. Valvular *stenosis* means that the valves, usually the aorta or *pulmonary* valves within the heart, are narrowed so that the smooth flow of blood is obstructed by the constriction. All of these defects put an extra work load on the heart. Tetralogy of Fallot is the name given a combination of defects causing a **blue baby**: "a ventricular septal opening; an 'overriding aorta' that straddles both ventricles instead of originating solely in the left ventricle; a stenosed pulmonary valve; and an enlarged right ventricle" (20).

Symptoms of congenital heart disease may show up at varying ages, usually in the early years. Blueness, failure to grow and gain weight, fatigue, and breathlessness may be present in some instances and not in others. Inborn heart defects account for one percent of all the heart diseases in adults.

The exact cause of inborn heart defects is still unknown. A small percentage may result from the mother having had German measles during the first trimester of pregnancy. Other outside influences may lead to imperfect development of the human embryo including the heart. Women who are pregnant should not take drugs or medicines without consulting their physicians.

Varicose Veins

Varicose or swollen *veins* are usually found on the inner side and back of the calf muscle of the leg and on the inner side of the thigh. They are blue and visible through the skin as it is the surface veins that are seriously damaged by varicosities.

Veins are low pressure blood vessels with less muscle tissue than arteries that carry blood back to the heart aided by valves which prevent the back flow of blood. Varicose veins are veins that have become stretched under pressure and the valves of which lose their efficiency and allow some back flow of blood.

There is probably an inherited weakness in the structure of veins of people who suffer from varicosities. The environmental factors which may bring about a change in structure are many. The most common being abdominal pressure that comes during pregnancy resulting from the enlarging uterus and increased blood flow to and from the abdominal and pelvic areas which act indirectly to hinder the flow of blood from the legs. Heavy lifting and straining may cause such pressure. As one ages the loss of the tone of tissue around the veins occurs with resulting loss of support. Obesity most likely overworks the veins.

People in jobs that require prolonged standing may develop varicosities. Dentists, barbers, beauticians, and teachers seem to have a higher incident of this disability than do people in sitting down jobs. People in sitting jobs have a higher risk of varicose veins if it requires sitting for long periods of time. Tight clothing such as garters and girdles may interfere with the return of blood to the heart and thus increase the pressure on the veins.

People in certain jobs can seek relief by walking and getting their feet up in the air when sitting. Bicycling exercises, walking, and swimming are good exercises for persons with mild varicosities.

Besides the obvious change in appearance varicose veins become manifest by increased fatigue of the leg muscles, muscular cramps at night, soreness of the veins in the calf after prolonged standing and burning and itching sensations of the varicosities.

Treatment of mild cases of varicose veins is often successful by use of support hosiery. The hosiery supports the veins. Stockings for women and socks for men should be fitted carefully. The new stretch yarns have made hosiery a most effective means of therapy.

Injections of a sclerosing solution is sometimes used to block off the damaged part of the vein, the blood being rerouted through other vessels. Surgery for removing the vein or tying it off is usually more effective and the risk is slight. The physician must decide which if either of these two methods is advisable.

Most of this material on varicose veins was selected from Public Health Service Publication No. 154 (21). The reader should note that other references of this kind are used frequently. These publications can be secured in single copies by writing the National Institute of Health, Bethesda, Maryland, 20014.

Transplants

In recent years the sensational news about heart disease has been transplants of the whole organ. Ulys H. Yates, medical science writer for the American Medical Association (22) points out that these are not spectacular leaps into "futuristic medicine" but the result of years of continuing research and clinical study. He also points out that such transplantations will be useful to only a limited number of patients, those older people who suffer from *congestive* heart failure or infants born with defects so severe they cannot live. People who suffer from coronary heart disease are not patients to receive transplants as atherosclerosis is not an immediate threat to life.

Heart transplants are limited for several reasons. Donors are not easily available because the heart is often affected by the injury or disease from which they die and many of those whose heart could be used do not die at a time or place so that use is possible. Also, much more research into the immune reaction is necessary. The body of the recipient builds *antibodies* attached to small lymphocytes and after a period of time these destroy the transplanted organ. This action can be suppressed somewhat by chemicals but at the risk of lowering the resistance to infection. *Antiserums* are being experimented with in kidney transplants and research in other aspects of this rejection process continues. As Yates notes in the long run "the major questions and problems regarding organ transplantations may be not medical but ethical, legal, and moral considerations" (22, p. 37).

The transplantation of segments of veins, arteries, bones, and tendons and the cornea of the eye are relatively easy because they do not need a copious blood supply and so are not seriously troubled by the rejection process.

The use of artificial devices may hold as much promise as that of transplants. Crimped Dacron and Teflon tubes are widely used to replace blood vessels and to serve as bypass grafts to route blood around diseased or obstructed blood vessels in some types of stroke, *renal* hypertension and closed vessels of the extremities. Artificial heart valves and *pacemakers* have been used successfully for several years. The development of such devices is advancing rapidly and the time may come soon when they will be used as substitutes for whole organs. Though they may never function as well as transplanted organs they can be easily obtained and will not be rejected by the host (23).

BIBLIOGRAPHY FOR HEART DISEASE

1. DAWBER, T. R.; KANNEL, W. B.; REVOTSKIE, N.; STOKES, J.; KAGAN, A.; GORDON, T., "Some Factors Associated with the Development of Coronary Heart Disease. Six Years Follow-up Experience in the Framingham Study." *American Journal of Public Health.* 49 (1959), p. 1349-1356.
2. *Reduce Your Risk of Heart Attack.* New York City: American Heart Association, 44 East 23rd Street. 1966.
3. STAMLER, JEREMIAH, M.D.; DAVID M. BERKSON, M.D.; HOWARD A. LINDBERG, M.D.; YOLANDA HALL, M.S.; WILDA MILLER, M.P.H.; LOUISE MOJONNIER, PH.D.; MONTE LEVINSON, M.D.; DONALD B. COHEN, M.D.; QUENTIN D. YOUNG, M.D., "Coronary Risk Factors." *The Medical Clinic of North America.* Reprint, 50 (January 1966), p. 229-254.
4. STARE, FREDERICK J. "Over-nutrition," *American Journal of Public Health.* 53 (November 1963), p. 1795-1803.
5. STAMLER, JEREMIAH, *Lectures on Preventive Cardiology.* New York: Grune and Stratton, Inc., 1967.

6. MORRIS, J. N. and MARGARET D. CRAWFORD, "Coronary Heart Disease and Physical Activity of Work," British Medical Journal (December 20, 1958), pp. 1485-96.
7. JOHNSON, MARY LOUISE, BERTHA S. BURKE, and J. MAYER, "Relative Importance of Inactivity and Overeating in the Energy Balance of Obese High School Girls," American Journal of Clinical Nutrition, IV (January-February, 1956).
8. CUSHMAN, WESLEY P. and BRUCE L. BENNETT, Selected Health Problems. Columbus, Ohio: Charles E. Merrill Publishing Company, 1967.
9. MATHEWS, DONALD K., Beginning Conditioning. Belmont: Wadsworth Publishing Co., Inc., 1965.
10. Royal Canadian Air Force, Exercise Plans for Physical Fitness. New York: Pocket Books, Inc., 1962.
11. BLAKESLEE, ALTON and JEREMIAH STAMLER, M.D., Your Heart Has Nine Lives. New York: Pocket Books, Inc., 1963.
12. Smoking and Health, Report of the Advisory Committee to the Surgeon General of the Public Health Service, U. S. Government Printing Office, 1964.
13. KANNEL, WILLIAM B., M.D., Habits and Coronary Heart Disease, The Framingham Heart Study (Public Health Service Pamphlet No. 1515), U. S. Government Printing Office, 1966.
14. TOMKINS, SILMAN S., PH.D., "Psychological Model for Smoking Behavior" Supplement, American Journal of Public Health, 56 (December 1966), pp. 17-20.
15. HORN, DANIEL, PH.D., "Some Dimensions of a Model for Smoking Behavior Change," Supplement, American Journal of Public Health, 56 (December 1966), pp. 21-26.
16. "Want to Quit Smoking? Here are Tested Ways," Today's Health, 47 (May 1969), p. 84.
17. Epidemiology of Stroke, (Public Health Service Pamphlet No. 1607), U. S. Government Printing Office, 1967.
18. Cerebral Vascular Disease and Strokes, (Public Health Service Pamphlet No. 513), U. S. Government Printing Office, 1968.
19. Rheumatic Fever, (Public Health Service Pamphlet No. 144), U. S. Government Printing Office, 1967.
20. Inborn Congenital Heart Defects, (Public Health Service Pamphlet No. 1204), U. S. Government Printing Office, 1968.
21. Varicose Veins, (Public Health Service Pamphlet No. 154), U. S. Government Printing Office, 1966.
22. YATES, ULYS H., "Transplanation Today and Tomorrow," Today's Health, 46 (April 1968), pp. 33-38.
23. Fact Sheet: Artificial parts for the heart and blood vessels. National Health Institute. United States Public Health Service, 1967.

1. Evidence indicates that overweight people suffer from more maladies than do those victims within the 'normal' weight range. How would you define 'overweight'? What is the difference between overweight and obesity?
2. Which do you feel would be the more hazardous course: (a) to gain 30 excess pounds at age 23, and maintain the new level for the next forty years; or (b) to gain 20 excess pounds at age 23, and then fluctuate back and forth between 'normal' and plus twenty over the next forty years? Explain.
3. If a person cuts down his daily diet by one slice of buttered bread per day and kept all other factors constant, how much weight might he lose in a year?
4. What criteria would you establish for a college graduate who wants to maintain his 'playing weight'? Why is body weight sometimes a misleading statistic in evaluating one's level of fitness?
5. What effects does exercise really have on your cardiovascular system?
6. Why do you think the heart attack rate among males is higher than it is among females (up to age 65)? Do you have any reasons to suspect this trend will change in the future?
7. How does the smoking of cigarettes affect your cardiovascular system? If you smoked two packages of cigarettes a day, which would be more harmful, chain smoking, or spaced smoking? Why?
8. Hypertension is instrumental in a considerable number of heart diseases. What causes this hypertension? How can it be reduced (a) by the individual himself; (b) by medical attention?
9. If heart transplants ever do become 'perfected', will people still suffer from cardiovascular disorders with their "new" heart? Explain.

CHAPTER 2

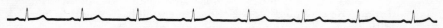

Cancer

Cancer, like heart disease, is not a single disease entity. Malignant tumors or cancers are divided into two main classes: *carcinomas* which develop in the lining and covering tissues of the organs; and *sarcomas* which develop in the connective and supportive tissues of the body. The word cancer is used to cover all malignancies and the basic principles of prevention and control that need be understood by the layman hold for all types.

Malignant tumors differ from *benign* tumors in that the latter grow locally and have more or less fixed borders which can be identified. Malignant tumors or cancers are characterized by a wild growth of functionless cells which invade adjacent tissue and spread to other areas of the body through the lymphatic and circulatory systems.

It is this ability of cancer cells to break off (*metastasize*) and form new colonies of cells elsewhere that makes the disease so treacherous. Because *metastasis* may come very early in the new growth (*neoplasm*) two steps in our cancer risk reduction program are related to early detection. They are: heed the seven danger signals and have periodic medical examinations. The third step is avoid cancer producing agents.

Heed the Seven Danger Signals

Cancer is a wild growth of cells which cause damage by compressing, invading and destroying contiguous normal tissue. Cancer cells are not *phagocytic* cells but destroy normal cells by depriving them the opportunity for normal nutrition and function. The danger signals are easy to remember if one understands the process.

1. *A lump or thickening that persists especially in the breast, lip, tongue, armpit or groin* should be suspected of being malignant until proven otherwise. The breast is a common site of cancer in women, yet only one of twenty growths on the breast are malignant. The most common type of breast cancer is a gland and if discovered while still small is curable. Such growths can be found by a monthly self-examination of the breast. If the growth is malignant and not detected early

metastasis may occur. Cells that break off pass from the primary site and set up a secondary growth elsewhere. This site may be a *lymph* gland, that is why lumps in the armpit or groin should be checked out. Cancer of the breast most often spreads to the armpit but may also reach the lungs. Cancer of the lip is most common among pipe smokers and the growth usually occurs at that point where the smoker holds his pipe and where the tissue of the lip joins the skin. A lump on the tongue or cheek may result from a chronic irritation caused by a broken tooth, poorly fitting dentures, or smoking.

2. *Bleeding from any normal body opening* may result from a break down in the blood vessels at the site of the malignancy. For example, blood in the stool of a person may appear from cancer in the colon or rectum, bloody *sputum* may be a signal of lung cancer. Blood from the vagina might lead one to suspect a malignancy of the uterus, but too often a woman may delay going to her physician believing that the bleeding is "only an irregularity in her menstrual flow." This is unfortunate because the "wait and see" period may be just long enough to allow the cancer to metastasize through the lymphatic system to glands within the pelvis or through the blood system to more distant organs. Blood in the urine may be a sign of cancer of the bladder. It should be noted that blood from a normal body opening may be a sign of difficulties other than a malignant tumor. This is true of all the other danger signals; but when the cause of these signs is unknown medical diagnosis should be sought.

3. When cancer cells invade normal tissue *a sore that does not heal* may occur. These noticeable sores appear particularly on the lips, tongue, ears, eyelids, or genital organs.

4. *Persistant hoarseness or cough* may be a sign of cancer of the throat or larynx. The most common early symptom of laryngeal cancer is a prolonged hoarseness which results from a tumor on the vocal cords. If growths occur elsewhere on the larynx they may cause voice change, "lump in the throat feeling," pain in swallowing or coughing.

Early detection of the site of the malignancy is most important for successful treatment. If detected early, in 2/3 or more of the cases the patient is able to retain the larynx. Fortunately, symptoms appear early; unfortunately, their mildness is often misleading and they are not heeded until too late.

5. *Persistent indigestion* is a sign often listed as a danger signal. Unfortunately, this symptom is often mild and vague so is shrugged off as "something I ate." If stomach pain or digestive discomfort continue more than two weeks no matter how vague or mild, a doctor should be consulted. The other signs which would probably be heeded such as blood in the stool, vomiting, and loss of weight, may not appear until twenty months after the malignant tumor has been present. By then a secondary tumor may be developing in the liver or adjacent lymph glands.

6. After one reaches forty, any marked *change in bowel habits* should be viewed with suspicion. A person with constipation or diarrhea that persists more than two weeks should see their physician. Feelings of incomplete evacuation may remain after a bowel movement. Only occasionally does abdominal discomfort or pain occur before metastasis. Unfortunately, advertising has made many Americans believe they are experts when it comes to treating constipation.

7. *A change in the size of warts or moles* is the last of our seven danger signals. *Melanoma*, which spreads rapidly, forms in some moles that are subject to irritation and in special locations such as the sex organs and feet. Most moles are not malignant nor will they become so. The average person has thirty or more moles over his body which have a genetic origin and appear off and on throughout his life time. Moles may darken after exposure to the sun, during puberty and pregnancy. After a person reaches middle age he may acquire *pigmented* areas that are not moles but wart-like growths that appear to have been stuck on the face or trunk or multiple brown spots on the wrists, back of hands, forearms and face (1). The vast majority of moles and blemishes are benign. The ones that warrant medical attention are those that bleed, itch, become painful, as well as suddenly change in size, and shape.

Medical Examinations

Periodic medical examinations are most important in the control of cancer for they can lead to early detection. Every good physician keeps the possibility of cancer in mind as he annually examines his patients particularly those over thirty. Examinations that have proven worthwhile in symptomless individuals include a general physical inspection and *palpation* of the whole body, with special attention to the cavities of the mouth, the vagina, the bladder, and the rectum. The vaginal smear test (Pap) for cervical cancer should be a routine annual procedure on all women of adult age. If women had such a test the mortality for uterine cancer could be cut by ninety percent.

In making an oral examination the physician may use a laryngeal mirror. This long handled mirror can enable the physician to detect most tumors of the larynx. He will, of course, look for lumps and sores on the tongue, lips, and cheeks. He will also check for a precancerous condition known as *leukoplakia* that tends to become malignant. Leukoplakia is a painless white patch of cells that forms on the tongue and mouth lining which may disappear if the source of irritation is removed, i.e.: smoking, broken teeth. A dentist routinely checks his patients for signs of oral cancer during their periodic visits.

A simple *rectal* examination can be performed that may lead to the discovery of cancer of the prostate gland, bladder or colon. The physician, by inserting his finger into the anal opening can feel many times the tumors that occur in the rectum. If a bladder tumor is large, it can sometimes be detected during a rectal or vaginal examination. *Prostate* cancer causes few deaths under forty; but after fifty it becomes the third highest cause of cancer deaths among men. The initial step in detecting the cancer is a rectal examination. The physician can feel irregular or unusually firm areas that may indicate a tumor. Fortunately, prostate cancer tends to be slow in metastasizing and growth usually begins in the back of the gland where it can be felt.

As indicated above there are no early signs of lung cancer, periodic chest X-rays may be helpful in finding a lung malignancy early enough for successful treatment. Periodic chest X-rays are, of course, valuable for other reasons.

Periodic examinations will not detect all cancers. Many procedures that could be used on a routine basis are used only where symptoms are present because they are uneconomical in terms of time, discomfort, and being hazardous to the patient. For example, a routine check that involves no risk to the patient and a minimum of discomfort is a *proctosigmoidoscopic* examination of the rectum and *colon*. This examination is recommended annually for all persons over forty years of age and unquestionably can frequently detect tumors before symptoms develop when prompt treatment can be most effective. As a general procedure the recommendation has but little chance of being adopted by many people because it requires a specialist who often practices in another part of town for whom an appointment must be made weeks in advance, because it involves a fee which though not unreasonable by medical standards, seems high to the patient and because even a little discomfort is often dreaded. Add these "becauses" to the patients underlying fear that "they might find something" and you have a screening practice that will not be widely accepted.

Avoid Carcinogens

Avoid *carcinogens* is the third and last step in the cancer risk reduction program. Carcinogens are the agents that cause cancer. And though how cancer is caused is not known, a causal relationship between certain cancers and certain agents has been well established through biostatistics, clinical evidence and laboratory experiments. The evidence provides us with information as to the specific agents to avoid.

Perhaps the best example from the personal health point of view is to avoid the agents contained in tobacco smoke. The Surgeon General's report on Smoking and Health states, "Cigarette smoking is causally related to lung cancer in men; the magnitude of the effect of cigarette smoking far outweighs all other factors. The data for women, though less extensive, point in the same direction" (2, p. 196). If one accepts this as the best evidence we have to date he should act on it. As can be gleaned from our discussion above there are no early signs of lung cancer. Only 5 percent of malignant lung tumors will produce blood streaked sputum the symptom that is apt to send the person to his doctor. The other symptoms are so commonplace they rarely send a patient to his physician. Early diagnosis is difficult even with annual X-rays and consequently is rare. Persons who do not smoke cigarettes reduce the risk of cancer of the lungs by 80 percent or more and even after years of smoking a person who stops improves his chances of not having the disease. Cancer of the bladder may not show early signs and smoking may be a causal factor. The present explanation is that smoking reduces the ability of the body to break down tryptophan. Some of the incomplete products of this *amino acid* are known cancer causing agents. These substances collect in the bladder. Laboratory studies show a marked increase in the amount of these carcinogens in the urine of cigarette smokers (3).

Avoiding smoking and heavy drinking reduces the risk of laryngeal cancer. Case histories reveal few men with cancer at this site who are not heavy smokers and/or drinkers. A British study showed that bartenders and tobacconists have significant higher rate of cancer than the general population. An American study showed that very few Seventh Day Adventists were admitted to hospitals with cancer of the larynx. Smoking and drinking among people of this religion is rare (4).

Though self-pollution of the air one breathes by smoking cigarettes is most significant, there is evidence to show that chemicals from industrial wastes, automobile exhausts and household sources are also factors in causing cancer. City dwellers have about 3 times more lung cancer than rural inhabitants. Reducing the risk of cancer from such sources is a community health problem. It must be solved by citizens, industry, local, state and the federal governments working hand and hand. In 1963 Congress enacted the Clean Air Act which provides for a national program for the prevention and control of air pollution. State governments are also initiating programs. If citizens act to finance such legislation this problem can be solved.

There are hundreds of chemicals that humans are exposed to through industry. Dye workers that handle betanaphthylamine run the risk of cancer of the bladder; workers who inhale or ingest radium increase the risk of bone cancer, people working with the chromates and asbestos risk lung cancer while those handling distillation and fractionation of coal and petroleum expose themselves to cancer of the skin. Industry acts to protect the worker against these carcinogens once they are identified but such protection is not a simple matter. It takes a period of years of continual exposure to the agent before cancer manifests itself, there is often a turnover in workers, and new chemicals are being developed and used so longitudinal studies are difficult to pursue (5, p. 50).

Light-complected people should avoid excessive exposure to the sun, the leading cause of skin cancer. Anyone can develop this disease but fair, ruddy or sandy complexioned people are more susceptible. This is probably because their skin lacks melanin which filters out the harmful ultraviolet rays of the sun (6).

Exposure to radiation is not a cause for great concern. The Division of Radiological Health of the Public Health Service has surveillance networks all over the country to determine current radiation levels in our environment including air, water, milk, and food. It is also cooperating with interested groups to help state and local authorities develop or improve radiological safety programs. However, as about 85 percent of man's exposure to man-made radition are medical ones it is recommended that individuals and their physicians keep records of X-ray and fluorscopic examinations and radiation treatments.

Viruses and Cancer

Cancer develops from changes in normal cells. There are three principles that govern normal growth: cell division, cell differentiation, and control of division. From the original fertilized egg there develops a community of some 100 billion cells that make up the individual. Each cell has the same genetic quality of the parent cell but some are different than others because of specialization to function as bone, muscles, liver, or brain cells. When sexual maturity is reached growth ceases and cell division serves a repair and replacement function. If tissue is injured destroying some of the cells, the remaining cells divide and multiply enough, but only enough, to repair the damage. Control is a property of normal cell division. In cancer, for reasons unknown, normal cells lose their function and control.

Cancer cells resemble the normal organ tissue from which they originate though they may be somewhat larger and abnormal in shape. Many cancers form glands and secrete the substances as the glands from which they arise. For example, tumors of the pituitary gland may secrete too much growth hormone so the patient shows a thickening of the bones of the hands and jaw. But control is missing and the cancer cells continue to divide, invade and compress and may metastasize to begin a new growth elsewhere.

There are three classes of agents that can cause cancer, two of which have been repeatedly mentioned in our discussion of risk reduction measures, chemicals and radiant energy. The third is viruses.

Peyton Rous of the Rockefeller University in New York demonstrated that a virus plays a role in one type of malignant tumor. But at the time, 1911, researchers were preoccupied with the bio-chemical role of the polycyclic hydrocarbons and genetic factors. Few scholars were interested in virus studies.

Studies by scientists showing that the concept of a specific virus as the cause of a specific tumor was false, studies developing better means for working with viruses such as growing viruses on tissue cultures and observing them by the means of the electron microscope, and the development of various techniques for identifying them renewed the interest of researchers in virus-cancer studies during the mid-fifties. Experiments with laboratory animals have definitely linked *leukemia,* cancer of the blood forming organs, to viruses and various findings contribute to the suspicion that viruses cause some forms of human cancer.

The findings have been such that today many scientists feel it is no longer a question of whether viruses can cause human cancer but what cancers are due to what viruses, and what are the mechanics involved? According to Dr. Michael B. Shimkin (5, p. 68) it is reasonable to postulate that permanent changes in the DNA (desoxyribonucleic acid) or RNA (ribonucleic acid) of a cell can be brought about by chemicals and by physical energy as well as by viruses, and that it is not necessary at this time to restrict the carcinogenic stimuli to any one class of agents, viruses or otherwise. If viruses are a cause of some cancer, it is possible that vaccines may be developed to build resistance to them. It is also possible that certain of these may be infectious. But we still can be sure that human cancer is not communicable, that is, that patient with cancer cannot pass it on to another human by direct or indirect contact.

There are many variables in the development of cancer. Chemicals, viruses, radiation or combinations of these (co-carcinogens) may initiate changes in normal cells that cause them to multiply wildly. An inherited susceptibility to certain cancers by individuals is a distinct possibility. Research is moving rapidly in many directions and the answers may soon be forthcoming. In the meantime, the college student has much to gain by following the risk reduction program previously outlined: heed the danger signals, have periodic medical examinations and avoid carcinogens.

Diagnosis and Treatment

A diagnosis of cancer cannot be definitely made without a biopsy. In this surgical procedure, "a small piece of suspect tissue is removed, placed in a preservative, cut in very thin slices, placed on a glass slide, stained with special dyes, and examined under the microscope." (7, p. 6) From our previous discussion, it is obvious that in certain instances to obtain a sample of tissue from internal tumors such as those of the lungs, stomach, colon and bone, surgery must be performed. Biopsy must not be confused with the previous mentioned cytological test for uterine cancer, the "Pap" smear. This technique named after its developer, Dr. George N. Papanicolaou, involves a microscopic examination of cells scraped from the cervix or collected in the fluid from the vagina. This procedure is being used to examine body fluids such as urine, sputum, washing from the stomach and smears from the nose and mouth. Cell tests such as these are useful in finding early cancer and aiding in diagnosis but only a biopsy provides a definite diagnosis of cancer.

Effective treatment of cancer depends on early diagnosis. If the cancer is detected before it metastasizes, surgery or radiation can be used with a most favorable prognosis. A person is considered cured if there is no recurrence of the malignancy within a five year period.

Surgery is the most effective way of curing operable cancer. In surgery, usually some normal tissue surrounding the site of the malignancy is cut out to be sure that all the disease is removed. New ways for preventing surgical shock and new drugs to prevent infections, plus new tools such as laser beams and ultra-sonic waves have made surgery more and more successful.

X-rays and radiation destroy cancer cells much more quickly than they do normal cells. In treatment the trick is to kill the malignant cells without too much damage to the normal tissue. New techniques for directing radiation on specific tissue and the development of radioactive substances which can be placed within the body are improving the effectiveness of such treatment.

Except in isolated instances cure of cancer through chemotherapy has not been accomplished. It is not difficult to find chemicals that will destroy cancer cells but it is difficult to find chemicals that will select only cancer cells for destruction and not destroy the normal cells a person needs to live. Research is difficult because cancer tissue varies and chemicals that impede cancerous growth in laboratory animals may show no effect on human cancer. Except for some individuals with terminal cancer human volunteers are hard to come by. In spite of the difficulties faced by researchers several groups of agents have been found to be helpful. Chemotherapy is used to block cell growth in a number of ways: *antimetabolites* are used to shut down the prolific multiplication of cancer cells; *cytotoxic* agents exhibit a tendency to destroy cancer cells in preference to normal cells; hormones seem to suppress some of the symptoms of cancer in some of the sex organs and in acute lymphocytic leukemia; chemicals such as iodine and phosphorous which certain parts of the body normally pick up if given in radioactive form (radioactive isotopes) will tend to irradiate against the cancers located in those organs which absorb them. An *antigen* is a substance which stimulates the formation of an *antibody*. Viruses are antigenic and build immune responses. When scientists are able to isolate specific viruses that cause cancer it may be possible to develop vaccines that can produce an active immunity against certain malignancies. Drugs other than anticancer drugs are used in the treatment of patients to relieve symptoms and ease pain and discomfort (8).

BIBLIOGRAPHY — CANCER

1. *Common Sense About Moles,* Committee on Cutaneous Health and Cosmetics, Chicago, Illinois: American Medical Association, 1968.
2. *Smoking and Health,* Report of the Advisory Committee to the Surgeon General of the Public Health Service, U. S. Government Printing Office, 1964.
3. *Cancer of the Bladder,* (National Institute of Health Publication No. 29), U. S. Government Printing Office, 1968.
4. *Cancer of the Larynx,* (Public Health Service Publication No. 1284), U. S. Government Printing Office, 1965.

1. Cancer, detected early, can be cured. Why is it that this disease is generally not caught in its earliest stages?
2. Why do you think people are so reticent about going to the doctor for a medical checkup?
3. If cigarette smoking really does cause cancer, why is it that smoking women have a lower incidence of lung cancer than their male counterparts?
4. If a friend of yours told you he was sure he had cancer because he had a sore throat, a cough, and a swelling on his neck, how would you respond?
5. What are the most effective ways of treating cancer? What current research is underway in this field?

5. SHIMKIN, MICHAEL B., M.D., *Science and Cancer,* (Public Health Service Publication No. 1162), U. S. Government Printing Office, 1964.
6. *Cancer of the Skin,* (National Institute of Health Publication No. 28), U. S. Government Printing Office, 1968.
7. *The Cancer Story,* (Public Health Service Publication No. 1162-B), U. S. Government Printing Office, 1966.
8. *Drugs vs. Cancer,* (Public Health Service Publication No. 1652), U. S. Government Printing Office, 1967.

CHAPTER 3

Diabetes Mellitus

Diabetes mellitus is a risk in cardiovascular diseases. The relationship shows up clearly in the complications of the disease of which heart defects compose 21 percent, hypertension 17 percent, and impaired vision over 10 percent. In this country there are over 2.4 million people with this disease plus an estimated 1.6 million undetected cases (1, p. 120).

There are two types of diabetes, juvenile and adult. The juvenile is more severe and occurs most frequently during childhood and adolescence. Before the discovery of *insulin,* the disease progressed rapidly with hardening of the arteries in many areas of the body with resulting complications such as gangrene in the extremities, blindness, heart attacks, and kidney disease. Insulin controls this type but the life expectancy of the juvenile diabetic is shortened. The adult-type or maturity-onset diabetes which accounts for seventy percent of all cases is usually detected after 40 years of age and is less severe (2, p. 67); (3, p. 533).

As this discussion develops it will become apparent that much more needs to be known before we are even close to the methods of prevention and control of diabetes. Until the facts are in, the following risk reduction program is recommended: maintain normal weight; exercise regularly; heed the danger signals; have periodic medical check-ups.

Maintain Normal Weight

How to maintain normal weight has been discussed in some detail as a risk reduction step in heart disease. All authorities seem to agree that obesity is a risk factor in adult-type diabetes which appears usually after forty. Over 80 percent of these diabetics show a history of overweight before the onset of the disease (2, p. 533). The obese person eats more than he needs and the excess calories are stored as body fat. It has been theorized that overeating places a greater than normal demand on the pancreas for insulin which exceeds the gland's ability to produce the hormone and diabetes results (4). Evidence from recent studies indicate that diabetes may be "primarily a disease of the vas-

cular system and not simply a disorder of carbohydrate metabolism"
(2, p. 67). This is in variance with the concept that abnormal carbohydrate metabolism is the initial sign and that small blood vessel diseases
develop as diabetes progresses.

The risks of having diabetes is higher in women than in men. There
seems to be little difference before twenty-five but after that women
are more susceptible. After sixty the rate becomes about the same. The
usual explanation given relates to pregnancy, as the highest rate among
women is among married women who have children. Perhaps glandular
changes during pregnancy can affect the way starches and sugars are
used, but recent studies do not indicate this is so; a more likely explanation is that after the birth women continue to carry the excess fat tissue
they put on during pregnancy (2, p. 67).

Exercise Regularly

There is no specific evidence to show that exercise prevents diabetes,
but we do know that in moderate amounts, exercise helps to reduce
the sugar in the body and makes it easier to control body weight. Exercise is considered beneficial for diabetes, but the amount of exercise
should be uniform and planned in relation to the treatment prescribed
by the physician.

Heed the Danger Signals

The signs and symptoms of diabetes are easily remembered if one
has an elementary understanding of the physiological processes. In the
juvenile type of diabetes the disease manifests itself when the body
can no longer make use of carbohydrates in a normal way because of
the lack of insulin. In the adult onset type of diabetes the action of
the insulin is "interferred with or blocked from performing its primary
task of facilitating the entry of glucose (blood sugar) into the cells
of the body." (2, p. 67) When insulin is lacking or blocked the body
can no longer use or store the glucose. This means it accumulates in the
blood. The kidneys then work overtime to excrete the excess, this
requires more water from the body tissue increasing urination. The
water from the tissue must be replaced so the person is thirsty. Because
the cells cannot get the glucose they need the person becomes weak,
tired, and hungry. The cells then use body proteins and fats as their
sources for energy needs so the person loses weight. The signs of diabetes are excessive thirst, frequent urination, uncommon hunger, loss of
weight and itching. Unfortunately, they are not early signs and before
they appear damage may have been done.

Periodic Medical Check-ups

The physician during his routine health examination will include a
urinalysis. He places a sample of urine in a test tube, adding a special
solution, and boils the mixture. If there is a color change, sugar is

present. If the test is positive it does not necessarily mean that the person has the disease so the doctor takes a sample of blood from the finger or ear lobe and tests it for the amount of sugar. If the case is borderline he may perform a glucose tolerance test to learn how well the body handles a specific amount of sugar (5, p. 3). Successful treatment of diabetes may depend on early detection.

Heredity and Diabetes

Heredity seems to be a factor in diabetes. A few years ago it was thought to be inherited as a recessive characteristic according to Mendelian law. Today this mode of transmission is questioned (6). But that heredity is a factor is borne out by the fact that among identical twins the condition develops at about the same time. Perhaps as high as one out of four people carry the diabetic trait. Since a person may not know of a family history of the disease, carriers may marry without being aware of this risk.

Young people often worry about whether they should marry after they have read about the probabilities that a child may be diabetic. There is little point in worrying but a couple should carefully consider how this disease may affect their marriage. Before insulin most diabetic women could not have children because they were sterile. After insulin the diabetic women had a high risk of miscarriages or stillbirth. But today, with new knowledge and new medicines, a diabetic woman has an 85 percent chance of having a healthy baby with little risk to her own health. Even if her child inherits the disease it may not affect him until late in life and if it develops earlier he can control the disease and be a productive person. Couples should always have a premarital examination to determine how health factors may influence their marriage. Living with a diabetic will involve more responsibilities such as supervision and added medical costs, but diabetes, per se, need not be a barrier to happiness in the family.

Treatment

There is no cure for diabetes, but control of the disease is possible. Before 1922 a child or adult with diabetes had a life expectancy of five to ten years. The discovery of insulin by Banting and Best has changed that picture completely. The diabetic can learn to take a water solution of insulin which he injects under the skin of his arm, abdomen or thigh varying the spot from day to day. The amount of insulin being prescribed by the doctor depends on many variables such as the severity of the case, and the caloric needs of the patient. Juvenile-type diabetes occurring usually before 30 are insulin-dependent and insulin sensitive. That is the juvenile-type will develop diabetic coma if he does not receive insulin and small changes in the dosage of insulin may cause problems for the patient. The life expectancy of the juvenile diabetic is shortened because insulin, though it maintains the patient, does not prevent the complications which develop as a result of the atherosclerosis which may develop in many parts of the body. The adult-type cases are usually not insulin-dependent and not sensitive to insulin. Many of the adult-type that cannot be controlled by diet alone can be controlled by the use of oral compounds which can be taken by mouth. Some of these chemicals lower the blood sugar level by stimulating the production of insulin by the pancreas. Others perhaps interfere with the "block" action of insulin which does not allow the glucose entry into the body cells (2, 3, 4).

There are two possible crises that diabetics face: insulin reaction and diabetic coma. The former occurs when the balance between the amount of insulin taken, food intake and exercise is upset. The blood level of sugar may drop too fast if the diabetic has taken too much insulin, too little food, or been more active than usual. The symptoms are sweating, hunger, trembling and faintness; and in severe cases: talking thickly, staggering drunkenly and becoming unconscious. In diabetic coma, the other crisis, the body lacking insulin uses fat for its source of energy. When the fats are used for energy fatty acids are formed. These acids, when they become excessive, can poison the body leading to coma and death. Today coma is rare but can occur in the severely diabetic person who neglects his diet or fails to take his insulin. In any case, it is recommended that the diabetic person carry an identification card saying he has the disease. It should provide for addresses and telephone numbers of the patient and his doctor. It may also carry instructions as to what to do. Insulin shock can usually be helped by administering candy, orange juice, or sugar. Coma requires immediate medical attention. (5, p. 11, 16)

It should be noted that diabetes is on the increase in this country. People are living long enough to develop the adult type and children who develop it are now remaining alive and are able to bear children thus increasing the number of offspring who will inherit the tendency toward the disease (6, p. 2).

BIBLIOGRAPHY — DIABETES MELLITUS

1. FISHBEIN, MORRIS, M.D., "Portrait of Our Diabetics," *Medical World News*, 8 (November 10, 1967), p. 120.
2. LAMONT-HAVERS, RONALD W., M.D., "Surprising Findings About Diabetes," *Today's Health*, 46 (April, 1968), p. 66.
3. STONE, DANIEL B., M.D., "Treating the Diabetic Patient," *Current Medical Digest*, 35 (May, 1968), p. 533.
4. *You and Diabetes*, Kalamazoo, Michigan: The Upjohn Company, 1964.
5. *Facts about Diabetes*, New York: American Diabetes Association, Inc., 1966.
6. *Diabetes Control. A Public Health Program Guide.* (Public Health Service Publication No. 506), U. S. Government Printing Office, 1969.

1. What logic is there in the theory that body weight and diabetes are closely linked? How does this reasoning stand up when it is added that women between the ages of 25-60 are more susceptible to diabetes than are men of similar age?
2. What effect might diabetes have on a marriage relationship?
3. What are the causes and effects of insulin reaction and diabetic coma?
4. What are the advantages and hazards of diabetics participating in vigorous physical activity?

CHAPTER 4

Epilepsy, Allergies, and Arthritis

Research has provided evidence that if young people will follow certain habits of living they can reduce substantially the chances of premature death and disability from certain cardiovascular diseases and cancer, diseases which develop over a period of time and manifest themselves usually at mid-age or later. There are other noncommunicable diseases about which young people should be informed, diseases which can be controlled and in some cases prevented but for which risk reduction programs cannot be as clearly identified.

Epilepsy

Epilepsy is a sign of some disorder of the brain. *Neurons,* nerve cells, of which there are millions in the brain, become overactive and discharge their electrical impulses irregularly. If the disturbance spreads it overwhelms the brain and a *seizure* results. Soon the neurons begin to work together again and the attack is over. The seizure is a sign of an abnormal release of energy in the brain. A diagnosis is made by use of an *electroencephalogram* which measures the brain waves.

Research within the last twenty-five years has made great advances in the control of the disease and an understanding of the nature of the trouble. It is estimated that perhaps one out of every two hundred people may have epilepsy with repeated seizures, but with today's medicines, eighty-five percent of these can live normal lives. With good medical care 50 percent of them become entirely free of seizures and another 30 percent will have their seizures well controlled. There are several varieties of seizure activity depending on the portion of the brain involved.

Grand mal (great sickness) seizures are often begun with an aura or warning in the form of a sigh, gasp, or cry. The patient loses consciousness and falls. He may clench his teeth and in so doing bite his tongue, he stiffens his body and may hold his breath after which there is a rhythmic hard jerking of the body. He may lose control of his bladder or bowels. He is in no serious danger unless he has fallen where he may hurt his head as he thrashes around. For a few minutes after the spell he may remain unconscious.

The petit mal (little sickness) may be characterized by blinking, pursing or licking of the lips, nodding the head, and a brief motionless stare. Such seizures may occur frequently throughout the day.

Psychomotor epilepsy is the most common type of a variety referred to as *focal*. Focal types are so called because the abnormal electrical discharges can be traced to a specific small area of the brain. In grand mal and petit mal the disordered release of energy spreads over the entire brain. In psychomotor seizures the discharging cells act upon the mental process as well as the muscles, resulting in bizarre behavior which usually lasts only a few minutes and is not remembered. The person unknowingly may kick, crawl, hit someone or cause property damage. One such case was detected because the boy could not explain why he knocked the lamps off the table and emptied the bookcases on the floor. In Jacksonian epilepsy, a focal type, seizures begin in the toes of the foot or fingers of one hand or in the corner of the mouth. The affected part trembles or feels numb and as more neurons are involved the trembling or numbness marches upward. These signs may last for a few minutes and the person then loses consciousness and has a spell like that in grand mal.

Diagnosis of epilepsy is made by the physician through many observations and tests. Careful reporting of the seizures by the person, friends, parents, teachers and others is most important to the doctor. Blood count, urinalysis, X-rays of the skull and brain-wave tests will be performed. The electroencephalogram (EEG) will probably be the conclusive evidence for the diagnosis.

In the past the physician had only bromides and phenobarbital to use in treatment. Unfortunately, the former caused dullness and the latter drowsiness. Today some twenty-five drugs are being used effectively under the supervision of medical personnel. So many new drugs are coming on the market that the National Institute of Neurological Diseases and Blindness have set up a panel of experts "to help doctors classify patients and evaluate the usefulness of a given drug in a given type of epilepsy" (2, p. 16). How these drugs work is not known. It is thought that they do not work on the discharging neurons themselves but somehow keep the electrical disturbance from spreading to other neurons. Once scientists find out how, a cure may be forthcoming.

The epileptic's problems are social as well as physiological. For centuries ignorance and superstition has been associated with specific diseases. For many years state laws permitted committing the epileptic to state mental hospitals with the lunatics and idiots. He was not permitted a marriage license being classified with habitual drunkards, criminals and the insane. He could not obtain a driver's license. If a child, he may not have been permitted to go to school and if adult, a job was hard to find. Fortunately, health education is doing much to change this situation. Most statutes have been changed so no longer is the epileptic classified with criminals or the insane. He can get a marriage license. In most states he can get a driver's license with limitations if a physician certifies he has not had seizures during the past year. Insurance companies, however, will not issue him an automobile liability policy. Workmen's Compensation laws have been changed so employment of epileptics no longer exposes the employer to the risks of increased premiums. So employers are much more willing to hire the epileptic today than in the past. With the increased control of seizures most school authorities are accepting the epileptic child. But education of the public is slow and it will be some time before feelings of shame or fear are divorced from the word epilepsy.

To complete this discussion, two questions that young adults raise need to be answered. Is it all right for an epileptic to marry? What do you do if a person has an attack?

A great many people still believe heredity to be the chief cause of epilepsy. Authorities feel that 25 percent of the cases of epilepsy have a hereditary basis through some inherent weakness in the brain or nervous system which predisposes to the disease or a chemical make up that makes it easy for the neurons to fire off overactively. Disease, birth injuries, accidents and others produce the seizures if the tendency is inherited. The chance of an epileptic parent having an epileptic child is only one in forty and the chances are only one in seventy that the seizures will become chronic (1:16). Certainly the role of heredity is small particularly where the disease has been traced to injury. The answer to the marriage question is then, "Yes, if the seizures are controlled well enough so the person can take on the responsibilities that come with marriage, and if the future partner is completely informed of the situation" (2, p. 23).

Once a seizure begins there is nothing you can do to stop it. The epileptic will not need a physician unless he goes into a series of spells without regaining consciousness. He is not going to die during the attack. You should protect him from hurting himself, particularly his head, if he is thrashing around. His movements should not be checked. If necessary to move him away from obstacles slide him by grasping his clothing around the trunk. Place a folded handkerchief between his teeth to keep him from biting his tongue. Do this only if it can be done without using force. Loosen tight clothing, particularly around the neck. When he regains consciousness, let him rest. He will be able to tell you how you can help him. This is the first aid to be carried out for grand mal seizures. In petit mal there is nothing to do and in psychomotor seizures the person should be allowed to continue his activity without restraint.

Allergies

An allergy is an abnormal reaction of the body to a harmless foreign substance—usually a protein. Instead of building a resistance to the *allergen,* as the body would to a harmful bacteria or virus, it builds a sensitivity. The sensitivity is established when the tissues of the nose or bronchi, for example, develop antibodies to pollens, grasses, weeds, molds, dust, dander, drugs, feathers, various foods, plants, insect stings, and others. After the antibodies have been developed the tissue reacts to that specific allergen. Also at this time histamine may be released which causes dilation of the blood vessels, increased flow of secretions and local irritation. (4, 5, 6, 7).

Allergies plague some nineteen million people, two thirds of whom suffer from hay fever or asthma. Prolonged and repeated sneezing; red, swollen, teary eyes and itchy nose and eyes are characteristics of hay fever. Actual fever is not. The pollens of trees, grasses and weeds and molds are easily air-borne and the hay fever victim suffers only when his specific allergen is in the air. Those who are sensitive to tree pollen suffer in the spring; those sensitive to grasses suffer in the early summer; those sensitive to ragweed may suffer from spring to late fall. People who are allergic to house dust, dog or cat dander or other inescapable airborne material may suffer all year long. The degree of suffering varies with the amount of pollen in the air and the sensitivity of the person. Some people may develop complications such as chronic sinusitis, nasal polyps (growths) and asthma (4).

Asthma develops because of the sensitivity of the bronchial tissues. When the allergen is airborne the lining of the bronchial tubes swells, the secretions thicken. The muscles, particularly in the branch-like extension of the bronchial tree, fail to release or dilate thus making it most difficult for the victim to expel air. The characteristic wheezing, coughing, and gasping ensues. Children get asthma; also adults in every age, race and occupation. In asthma, as with most all allergies, there is usually a family history of sensitivity and usually the victim has suffered previous to his asthma from skin rashes, hives, or hay fever. The attacks occur most often at night and the squeezing of the chest and throat bring a fear of choking. Attacks of asthma, though distressing, are rarely fatal. Children, when under care, often recover permanently when they reach their teens. There are effective medicines that doctors can use to relieve the distress and to end long lasting attacks. The causes are the same as in hay fever. Recent research has dispelled the myth that asthma may be a psychosomatic disease (8, p. 28).

Hay fever and asthma are controlled by removing the cause so far as is practical and building up the patient's resistance. Avoiding the specific substance is the best way to control the allergy. For the patient or the doctor to discover the offending substance is not always easy. A careful history of when the attacks occur may reveal the agent. If this method gives no clue, the doctor may have to perform as many as thirty or forty skin tests. He does this by scratching a powder or solution made up of the allergen into the skin; if a red welt or wheal appears the test is positive. Some people may be allergic to several different substances. Once the causative agent is identified it may be possible to avoid it. Seasonal vacations and air conditioning may help but have their limitations. The purchase of the latter should be carefully investigated. If the agent is dander the family pet may have to go (4, 8).

In many instances avoiding the substance is impossible. The doctor, having identified the agent, may then suggest building an immunity to it. He can make up a series of graded injections. The solution will contain a minute amount of the allergen; this amount is increased in each injection until the body can tolerate larger doses without reaction. The injections have to be repeated annually though after several years desensitization to the specific substance may occur (4, 8). The availability of testing and desensitization is limited by the few specialists in the field.

The sticky sap of poison ivy, oak and sumac contains an active ingredient known as urushiol though this substance is not identical in each plant. In each, however, it causes allergic skin reactions. Seven out of ten persons may become sensitized to any of the three plants. The rash may be mild or severe, appear a few hours or several days after contact. The skin may turn red and itch or large blisters and swelling may appear depending on the sensitivity of the person and the degree of exposure. Avoiding the plants is the best preventive measure because urushiol must make contact with the skin for a reaction. Smoke may carry drops of the chemical and pets may rub up against the plants and pass the sap to a person indirectly. It is well to wear long sleeves and trousers in the woods and pastures and maybe in your own back yard as poison ivy and poison oak grow almost everywhere. There is little risk of developing scars unless there is a secondary infection. Spreading is not due to the discharge from the blisters, but from the original or a new contact. The best treatment is sudsing the skin and washing clothes that may be contaminated. Most cases disappear by themselves. Calamine lotion is a good drying agent and relieves itching. For severe cases a doctor should be consulted (9).

Hives is an allergy most often caused by drugs and food. It starts below the skin surface and manifests itself in red surface swellings not unlike large mosquito bites. Common foods that are involved are cows milk in children, eggs, wheat, nuts, strawberries and shell fish. Once a food, and it can be any food, is identified it can be avoided. The American Dietetic Association, 620 North Michigan Avenue, Chicago, has suggested allergy recipes for people sensitive to foods. Drugs, particularly *antibiotics*, such as penicillin, are being used more frequently than in the past so it is not surprising to find more people sensitive to them. A person who has had a reaction to a specific drug or *antitoxin* should be aware of the greater danger that may arise if the drug is used again, especially if it is injected. Such people should wear a medical identification tag or carry a warning card for the allergy risks with medicines (10, p. 428).

Arthritis

Most adults will at some time suffer from some form of arthritis. This term which means inflammation of the joint is used by lay people to refer to a variety of aches and pains involving connective tissue holding together the bones, organs, glands and other structures of the body. Rheumatoid arthritis and osteoarthritis are the most common, the latter occurring in the later years. Gout and collagen diseases are other forms. Rheumatism is also a general term commonly used to describe stiffness and aching pain. This group of diseases afflicts more people than all the victims of cancer, diabetes, heart trouble and tuberculosis combined yet little was being done to help these sufferers until the Arthritis and Rheumatism Foundation was founded in 1948. This organization and others have been able recently to point up the magnitude of this health problem with the result much new knowledge about the forms of the disease and new treatment of them is available (11, 12, 10).

Rheumatoid arthritis attacks three times as many women as men. It is the most crippling form of the rheumatic diseases and unfortunately most often strikes housewives and working women between the ages of twenty and thirty-five. As the arthritis symptoms seem to increase during menses and decrease during pregnancy, specialists hold to the theory that there is a link between rheumatoid arthritis and the endocrine glands. It would seem that it is a disorder of metabolism which is the sum of the physical and chemical processes of the body. Attacks cause pain and swelling of the joints, weakness, fatigue and stiffness especially in the morning (10, p. 390). These manifestations may last for weeks or months varying in intensity. Arthritis frequently hits after an illness and in young mothers after the first child. Fatigue from work is a contributing factor. Fear and worry can trigger the onset. The signs and symptoms listed above should be considered warning signals and a physician consulted. If neglected they may recur and progress to fusion of the joints (13). The best treatment of the disease includes different methods and techniques. Drugs, a balance of exercise, activity and rest prescribed carefully by a physician can prevent progress of the disease. Rest reduces the joint inflammation, exercise retains muscle and joint function and prevents the onset of deformity. Drugs prescribed by the physician may include aspirin, chloroquin, gold salts by injections, and cortisones (10, p. 391). There is no single drug or other method of treatment that will cure or relieve this form of arthritis. The advice of a skilled physician is absolutely essential.

Osteoarthritis is most common in the older years, 80 percent of the afflicted being over sixty. It is relatively mild, usually non-crippling and usually involves a weight-bearing joint. It is more common among women than men, afflicting to some degree eighty percent of women sixty years of age or older. Hormonal changes also seem to be a factor in the development of this form of arthritis. Overweight is considered to be a contributing factor. The signs and symptoms which indicate medical consultation are pain and stiffness in the lower back, knees and other joints, and tingling sensations in the finger tips. Despite the mildness of these symptoms X-rays may reveal severe changes in the spine, hips, and knees. Early diagnosis and treatment can prevent further damage reducing the risk of increased pain and deformity (13). Treatment consists of prescribing exercise and drugs (usually limited to aspirin). The patient is helped psychologically by insuring him that the disease is not crippling or immobilizing. The Arthritis and Rheumatism Foundation suggests these preventive steps for women (13):

1. Relax housekeeping standards somewhat.
2. Rest half way through your ironing.
3. Do housework by installments.
4. Ease up with the children.
5. Maintain normal weight.
6. Avoid cold and dampness.
7. Avoid strain and worry.

Women can often avoid their long hours of housework. Afflicted men often have to change their jobs.

Gout is a severe form of acute arthritis that is usually limited to one or two joints. Heat, redness, tenderness and pain reach a peak in several hours and may last days or weeks. The acute type recedes and the victim is well for a varying period of time. The chronic kind persists. As gout is caused by faulty uric acid chemistry it is not surprising to learn that it is treated with drugs which assist in the elimination of the acid (10, p. 329).

Collagen diseases are forms of arthritis that involve the connective tissues that support the body. Bursitis is the most common. It is an inflammation of the bursae which are located in joints as lubricating membranes where muscles slide over one another. The shoulder and knee bursae most often become inflamed. Inflammation may also affect tendons, and joint-supporting or muscle sheaths. Often low back pain may be caused by such an inflammation (10, p. 393).

The new emphasis on research as to the cause of arthritis and rheumatism is international and should bring us new knowledge as to prevention and treatment of these diseases.

BIBLIOGRAPHY — EPILEPSY, ALLERGIES, AND ARTHRITIS

1. POLLOCK, JACK H., "Will Yours Be a Normal Baby?" *Today's Health*. 36 (March 1958), pp. 16-21.
2. *Epilepsy—Hope Through Research*. Public Health Service Publication No. 938, U. S. Government Printing Office, 1964.
3. LEONHARD, JACQUELINE T., *Diagnosis Epilepsy—A Guide for Parents*. Parents Committee on Epilepsy, Cleveland Family Health Association, Inc., 3300 Chester Avenue, 1962.

1. What is the major difference between "grand mal" and "petit mal"?
2. How are allergies detected? How is the causative agent discovered?
3. Why is it that some people are pestered by allergies all year round, while others only suffer during certain specific seasons?
4. Your daughter's boyfriend has asked to speak with you alone. You're quite sure he wants your blessing on his intention to marry her. He's an epileptic. How will you respond to him?
5. While in epileptic seizure, the person may cause damage to public property—should he be held responsible?

4. *Hay Fever, The Facts.* National Tuberculosis and Respiratory Disease Association, 1740 Broadway, New York City.
5. "What is an Allergy?" *Science Digest.* 64 (August 1968), pp. 87-8.
6. UNGER, DONALD L., "The Sneezin' Season Is Here," *Today's Health.* 45 (July 1967), p. 3.
7. "Allergies Plague 19 Million," *Science Newsletter.* 88 (July 17, 1965), p. 42.
8. DUCAS, DOROTHY, "Winning the Battle Against Asthma," *Today's Health.* 45 (August 1967), pp. 28-32.
9. *Poison Ivy, Oak & Sumac,* Public Health Service Bulletin No. 1723, U. S. Government Printing Office, 1967.
10. *Today's Health Guide,* Edited by W. W. BAUER, M.D., Chicago: American Medical Association, 1965.
11. *Stop Arthritis,* The Arthritis and Rheumatism Foundation, 23 W. 45th St., New York 36, N.Y.
12. *Questions About Arthritis and Rheumatism,* The Arthritis and Rheumatism Foundation, 23 W. 45th St., New York 36, N.Y.
13. *It's Women 3 to 1,* The Arthritis and Rheumatism Foundation, 23 W. 45th St., New York 36, N.Y.

Glossary

ACUTE — Having a sudden onset.

ADIPOSE — Relating to animal fat.

ALLERGEN — Any agent capable of producing an allergic reaction.

AMINO ACIDS — The chief chemical components of proteins.

ANEURYSM — A spindle-shaped or sac-like bulging of the wall of a vein or artery, due to weakening of the wall by disease or an abnormality present at birth.

ANGINA PECTORIS — Literally means chest pain. A condition in which the heart muscle receives an insufficient blood supply, causing pain in the chest, and often in the left arm and shoulder. Commonly results when the arteries supplying the heart muscle (coronaries) are narrowed by atherosclerosis. (1)

ANTIBIOTIC — An antibacterial substance produced by a living organism, such as fungus.

ANTIBODIES — A specific chemical protective substance formed in the body in response to the stimulation of an antigen.

ANTI-CARCINOGEN — An environmental agent offering some protection against a carcinogen similar in chemical construction.

ANTICOAGULENT — A drug which delays clotting of the blood. When given in cases of a blood vessel plugged up by a clot, it tends to prevent new clots from forming, or the existing clots from enlarging, but does not dissolve an existing clot. Examples are heparin and coumarin derivatives.

ANTIMETABOLITE — A closely similar but ineffective compound which tends to replace an essential cell building material.

ANTITOXINS — An antibody formed to neutralize a specific toxin.

ANTISERUMS — A serum containing antibodies.

AORTA — The main trunk artery which receives blood from the lower left chamber of the heart. It originates from the base of the heart, arches up over the heart like a cane handle, and passes

___

(1) Many of the physiological explanations of the heart and circulatory terms were taken from Health, Education, and Welfare, *A Handbook of Heart Terms* (Public Health Service Publication No. 1073).

down through the chest and abdomen in front of the spine. It gives off many lesser arteries which conduct blood to all parts of the body except the lungs.

AORTIC VALVE — Valve at the junction of the aorta, or large artery, and the lower left chamber of the heart. Formed by three cup-shaped membranes called semilunar valves, it allows the blood to flow from the heart into the artery and prevents a back flow.

APOPLEXY — Frequently called apoplectic stroke or simply a stroke. A sudden interruption of the blood supply to a part of the brain caused by the obstruction or rupture of an artery. Initially may be manifested by a loss of consciousness, sensation, or voluntary motion, and may leave a part of the body (frequently one side) temporarily or permanently paralyzed.

ARTERIOSCLEROSIS — Commonly called hardening of the arteries. This is a generic term which includes a variety of conditions which cause the artery walls to become thick and hard and lose elasticity.

ARTERY — Blood vessels which carry blood away from the heart to the various parts of the body. They usually carry oxygenated blood except for the pulmonary artery which carries unoxygenated blood from the heart to the lungs for oxygenation.

ATHEROSCLEROSIS — A kind of arteriosclerosis in which the inner layer of the artery wall is made thick and irregular by deposits of a fatty substance. These deposits (called atheromata) project above the surface of the inner layer of the artery, and thus decrease the diameter of the internal channel of the vessel.

AURICLE — The upper chamber in each side of the heart. "Atrium" is another term commonly used for this chamber.

BENIGN — Not malignant; not recurrent; favorable for recovery.

3, 4-BENZPYRENE — A chemical of a type known as polycyclic hydrocarbon that produces cancer in animals. It has been isolated from coal tar, and is found in the smoky atmosphere of industrial cities and the exhaust of internal combustion engines.

BETA-NAPHTHYLAMINE — A chemical of a type known as aromatic amine. It is a cause of bladder cancer among workers in aniline dye plants.

BICUSPID VALVE — Usually called mitral valve. A valve of two cusps or triangular segments, located between the upper and lower chamber in the left side of the heart.

BIOPSY — The removal and microscopic examination of tissue from the living body for purposes of diagnosis.

BLUE BABIES — Babies having a blueness of skin (cyanosis) caused by insufficient oxygen in the arterial blood. This often indicates a heart defect, but may have other causes such as premature birth or impaired respiration.

CALORIE — Sometimes called large or kilo-calorie. Unit used to express food energy. The amount of heat required to raise the temperature of 1 kilogram of water 1 degree Centigrade.
A high caloric diet has a prescribed caloric value above the total daily energy requirement. A low caloric diet has a prescribed caloric value below the total energy requirement.

CARCINOGEN — A cancer-causing agent.

CARCINOGENESIS — The production of cancer.

CARDIAC — Pertaining to the heart. Sometimes refers to a person who has heart disease.

CARDIOVASCULAR — Pertaining to the heart and blood vessels.

CELL — The basic unit of plant and animal life, consisting of a small mass of protoplasm, including a nucleus, surrounded by a semipermeable membrane.

CEREBRAL VASCULAR ACCIDENT — Sometimes called cerebrovascular accident, apoplectic stroke, or simply stroke. An impeded blood supply to some part of the brain, generally caused by one of the following four conditions:
1. a blood clot forming in the vessel (cerebral thrombosis)
2. a rupture of the blood vessel wall (cerebral hemorrhage)
3. a piece of clot or other material from another part of the vascular system which flows to the brain and obstructs a cerebral vessel (cerebral embolism)
4. pressure on a blood vessel as by a tumor

CEREBROVASCULAR — Pertaining to the blood vessels in the brain.

CHEMOTHERAPY — The treatment of disease by administering chemicals. Frequently used in the phrase "chemotherapy of hypertension," i.e., the treatment of high blood pressure by the use of drugs.

CHOLESTEROL — A fat-like substance found in animal tissue. In blood tests for normal level for American is assumed to be between 180 and 230 milligram per 100 cc. A higher level is often associated with high risk of coronary atherosclerosis.

CHROMOSOME — One of several small more or less rod-shaped bodies in the nucleus of a cell. The chromosomes contain the hereditary factors (genes) and are constant in number in each species.

CHRONIC — Always present, of long duration, not acute.

CIRCULATORY — Pertaining to the heart, blood vessels, and the circulation of the blood.

COAGULATION — Process of changing from a liquid to a thickened or solid state. The formation of a clot.

COARCTATION OF THE AORTA — Literally a pressing together, or a narrowing of the aorta which is the main trunk artery which conducts blood from the heart to the body. One of several types of congenital heart defects.

CO-CARCINOGEN — An environmental agent which acts with another to cause cancer.

COLLATERAL CIRCULATION — Circulation of the blood through nearby smaller vessels when a main vessel has been blocked up.

COLON — The large intestine.

CONGENITAL — Existing at birth.

CONGESTIVE HEART FAILURE — When the heart is unable adequately to pump out all the blood that returns to it, there is a backing up of blood in the veins leading to the heart. A congestion or accumulation of fluid in various parts of the body (lungs, legs, abdomen, etc.) may result from the heart's failure to maintain a satisfactory circulation.

CONSTRICTION — Narrowing, as in the phrase "vaso-constriction," which is a narrowing of the internal diameter of the blood vessels, caused by a contraction of the muscular coat of the vessels.

CORONARY ATHEROSCLEROSIS — Commonly called coronary heart disease. An irregular thickening of the inner layer of the walls of the arteries which conduct blood to the heart muscle. The internal channel of these arteries (the coronaries) becomes narrowed and the blood supply to the heart muscle is reduced.

CORONARY OCCLUSION — An obstruction (generally a blood clot) in a branch of one of the coronary arteries which hinders the flow of blood to some part of the heart muscle. This part of the heart muscle then dies because of lack of blood supply. Sometimes called a coronary heart attack, or simply a heart attack.

CORONARY THROMBOSIS — Formation of a clot in a branch of one of the arteries which conduct blood to the heart muscle (coronary arteries). A form of coronary occlusion.

CYTOTOXIC — Poisons cells.

DNA — (Deoxyribonucleic acid) — One of the two nucleic acids found in all cells. The other is RNA (ribonucleic acid). These exert primary control over life processes in all organisms.

DEFIBRILLATOR — Any agent or measure, such as an electric shock, which stops an incoordinate contraction of the heart muscle and restores a normal heart beat.

DIAGNOSIS — Act of identifying a disease.

DIASTOLE — In each heart beat, the period of the relaxation of the heart. Auricular diastole is the period of relaxation of the atria, or upper heart chambers. Ventricular diastole is the period of relaxation of the ventricles, or lower heart chambers.

DIET — Daily allowance or intake of food and drink.

DIGITALIS — A drug prepared from leaves of foxglove plant which strengthens the contract of the heart muscle, slows the rate of contraction of the heart, and by improving the efficiency of the heart, may promote the elimination of fluid from body tissues.

DUCTUS ARTERIOSUS — A small duct in the heart of the fetus between the artery leaving the left side of the heart (aorta) and the artery leaving the right side of the heart (pulmonary artery). Normally this duct closes soon after birth. If it does not close, the condition is known as patent or open ductus arteriosus.

EDEMA — Swelling due to abnormally large amounts of fluid in the tissues of the body.

ELECTROCARDIOGRAM — Often referred to as EKG or EGG. A graphic record of the electric currents produced by the heart.

ELECTROCARDIOGRAPH — An instrument which records electric currents produced by the heart.

ELECTROENCEPHALOGRAM — The tracing of brain waves made by an electroencephalograph.

EMBOLISM — The blocking of a blood vessel by a clot or other substance carried in the blood stream.

EMBOLUS — A blood clot (or other substance such as air, fat, tumor) inside a blood vessel which is carried in the blood stream to a smaller vessel where it becomes an obstruction to circulation.

EPIDEMIOLOGY — The science dealing with the factors which determine the frequency and distribution of a disease in a human community.

ESSENTIAL HYPERTENSION — Sometimes called primary hypertension, and commonly known as high blood pressure. An elevated blood pressure not caused by kidney or other evident disease.

ETIOLOGY — The sum of knowledge about the causes of a disease.

FIBRILLATION — Uncoordinated contractions of the heart muscle occurring when the individual muscle fibers take up independent irregular contractions.

GENETIC — Of, or pertaining to the genes, which are the biologic units of heredity located on the chromosomes.

HORMONES — Chemical products of the endocrine glands of the body which, when secreted into body fluids, have a specific effect on other organs.

HYPERCHOLESTEREMIA — An excess of a fatty substance called cholesterol in the blood. Sometimes called hypercholesterolemia or hypercholesterinemia.

HYPERTENSION — Commonly called high blood pressure. An unstable or persistent elevation of blood pressure above the normal range, which may eventually lead to increased heart size and kidney damage.

IMMUNITY — The body's ability to resist or overcome infection.

INFARCT — An area of a tissue which is damaged or dies as a result of not receiving a sufficient blood supply. Frequently used in the phrase "myocardial infarct" referring to an area of the heart muscle damaged or killed by an insufficient flow of blood through the coronary arteries which normally supply it.

INSUFFICIENCY — Incompetency. In the term "valvular insufficiency," an improper closing of the valves admits a back flow of blood in the wrong direction. In the term "myocardial insufficiency," inability of the heart muscle to do a normal pumping job.

INSULIN — A hormone secreted by the pancreas essential to the normal oxidation of sugar by the body cells.

INTIMA — The innermost layer of a blood vessel.

LARYNX — Voice box.

LESION — Any abnormal structural change in body tissues or organs.

LEUKEMIA — Cancer of the blood-forming organs, characterized by a marked increase of the blood elements known as leukocytes and their precursors.

LIPID — Fat.

LIPOPROTEIN — A complex of fat and protein molecules.

LUMEN — The passageway inside a tubular organ. Vascular lumen is the passageway inside a blood vessel.

LYMPH — A nearly colorless liquid composed of excess tissue fluid and proteins. Found in the lymphatic vessels of the body.

LYMPHOSARCOMA — A cancer arising in lymphatic tissue.

MALIGNANT — Tending or threatening to produce death.

MALIGNANT HYPERTENSION — Severe high blood pressure that runs a rapid course and causes damage to the blood vessel walls in the kidney, eye, etc.

MELANOMA — A skin tumor containing dark pigment.

MENSES — The menstruous flow.

METABOLISM — A general term to designate all chemical changes which occur to substances within the body.

METASTASIS (ES) — The transfer of disease from one part of the body to another. In cancer the new growths are characteristic of the original tumor.

METASTASIZE — To spread by metastasis.

MITRAL STENOSIS — A narrowing of the valve (called bicuspid or mitral valve) opening between the upper and the lower chamber in the left side of the heart. Sometimes the result of scar tissue forming after a rheumatic fever infection.

MITRAL VALVE — Sometimes called bicuspid valve. A valve of two cusps or triangular segments, located between the upper and lower chamber in the left side of the heart.

MURMUR — An abnormal heart sound, sounding like fluid passing an obstruction, heard between the normal lub-dub heart sounds.

MYOCARDIAL INFARCTION — The damaging or death of an area of the heart muscle (myocardium) resulting from a reduction in the blood supply reaching that area.

NEOPLASM — Any abnormal formation or growth, usually a tumor.

NEURONS — Nerve cells.

NUCLEUS — A specialized chromosome-containing portion of the protoplasm of cells. Coordinates the many cell activities.

OBESE — Excessively fat.

OPEN HEART SURGERY — Surgery performed on the opened heart while the blood stream is diverted through a heart-lung machine. This machine pumps and oxygenates the blood in lieu of the action of the heart and lungs during the operation.

PACEMAKER — A small mass of specialized cells in the right upper chamber of the heart which give rise to the electrical impulses that initiate contractions of the heart. The term "pacemaker," or more exactly, "electric cardiac pacemaker," or "electrical pacemaker" is applied to an electrical device which can substitute for a defective natural pacemaker and control the beating of the heart by a series of rhythmic electrical discharges.

PALPATION — Examination by touch.

PALPITATION — A fluttering of the heart or abnormal rate or rhythm of the heart experienced by the person himself.

"PAP SMEAR" — A technique developed chiefly by the late Dr. George N. Papanicolaou that involves the microscopic examination of cells collected from the vagina or other body cavity.

PATENT DUCTUS ARTERIOSUS — A congenital heart defect in which a small duct between the artery leaving the left side of the heart (aorta) and the artery leaving the right side of the heart (pulmonary artery), which normally closes soon after birth, remains open. As a result of this duct's failure to close, blood from both sides of the heart is pumped into the pulmonary artery and into the lungs. This defect is sometimes called simply patent ductus. Patent means open.

PHAGOCYTE — Devouring cell.

PHLEBITIS — Inflammation of a vein, often in the leg. Sometimes a blood clot is formed in the inflamed vein.

POLLENS — A mass of microspores in a seed plant.

POLYP — A mass of swollen mucous membrane projecting into the nasal or other cavity of the body.

POLY-UNSATURATED FAT — A fat so constituted chemically that it is capable of absorbing additional hydrogen. These fats are usually liquil oils of vegetable origin, such as corn oil or safflower oil. A diet with a high poly-unsaturated fat content tends to lower the amount of cholesterol in the blood. These fats are sometimes substituted for saturated fat in a diet in an effort to lessen the hazard of fatty deposits in the blood vessels.

PRIMARY HYPERTENSION — Sometimes called essential hypertension, and commonly known as high blood pressure. An elevated blood pressure not caused by kidney or other evident disease.

PROCTOSIGMOIDOSCOPE — A device for viewing the inside of the colon.

PROSTATE — The gland in the male that surrounds the urethra and the neck of the bladder.

PSYCHOSOMATIC — Pertaining to the influence of the mind, emotions, fears, etc. upon the functions of the body, especially in relation to disease.

PULMONARY ARTERY — The large artery which conveys unoxygenated (venous) flood from the lower right chamber of the heart to the lungs. This is the only artery in the body which carries unoxygenated blood, all others carrying oxygenated blood to the body.

PULMONARY VALVE — Valve, formed by three cup-shaped membranes at the junction of the pulmonary artery and the right lower chamber of the heart (right ventricle). When the right lower chamber contracts, the pulmonary valve opens and the blood is forced into the artery leading to the lungs. When the chamber relaxes, the valve is closed and prevents a back-flow of the blood.

PULMONARY VEINS — Four veins (two from each lung) which conduct oxygenated blood from the lungs into the left upper chamber of the heart (left atrium).

RADIUM — An intensely radioactive metallic element found in minute quantities in pitchblende and other uranium minerals. The radioactivity of radium is a result of disintegration of the atom.

RECTUM — Terminal part of the intestine.

REMISSION — A diminution or abatement of the symptoms of a disease; also the period during which such diminution occurs.

RENAL — Pertaining to the kidney.

RETINA — Sensory membrane of the eye that receives images.

RHEUMATIC FEVER — A disease, usually occurring in childhood, which may follow a few weeks after a streptococcal infection. It is sometimes characterized by one or more of the following: fever, sore swollen joints, a skin rash, occasionally by involuntary twitching of the muscles (called chorea or St. Vitus Dance) and small nodes under the skin. In some cases the infection affects the heart and may result in scarring the valves, weakening the heart muscle, or damaging the sac enclosing the heart.

RHEUMATIC HEART DISEASE — The damage done to the heart, particularly the heart valves, by one or more attacks of rheumatic fever. The valves are sometimes scarred so they do not open and close normally.

SATURATED FAT — A fat so constituted chemically that it is not capable of absorbing any more hydrogen. These are usually the solid fats of animal origin such as the fats in milk, butter, meat, etc. A diet high in saturated fat content tends to increase the amount of cholesterol in the blood. Sometimes these fats are restricted in the diet in an effort to lessen the hazard of fatty deposits in the flood vessels.

SCLEROSIS — Hardening, usually due to an accumulation of fibrous tissue.

SEDATIVE — A drug which depresses the activity of the central nervous system, thus having a calming effect. Examples are barbiturates, chloral hydrate, and bromides.

SEIZURE — A sudden attack, fit.

SEPTUM — A dividing wall.
1. Atrial or inter-atrial septum. Muscular wall dividing left and right upper chambers (called atria) of the heart.
2. Ventricular or inter-ventricular septum. Muscular wall, thinner at the top, dividing the left and right lower chambers (called ventricles) of the heart.

SIGN — Any objective evidence of a disease.

SPHYGMOMANOMETER — An instrument for measuring blood pressure in the arteries.

SPUTUM — Spit.

STENOSIS — A narrowing or stricture of an opening. Mitral stenosis, aortic stenosis, etc. means that the valve indicated has become narrowed so that it does not function normally.

STROKE — Also called apoplectic stroke, cerebrovascular accident, or cerebral vascular accident. An impeded blood supply to some part of the brain, generally caused by:
1. a blood clot forming in the vessel (cerebral thrombosis)
2. a rupture of the blood vessel wall (cerebral hemorrhage)
3. a piece of clot or other material from another part of the vascular system which flows to the brain and obstructs a cerebral vessel (cerebral embolism)
4. pressure on a blood vessel, as by a tumor.

SYMPTOM — Any subjective evidence of a patient's condition.

SYNDROME — A set of symptoms which occur together and are therefore given a name to indicate that particular combination.

SYSTOLE — In each heart beat, the period of contraction of the heart. Atrial systole is the period of the contraction of the upper chambers of the heart, called the atria.
Ventricular systole is the period of the contraction of the lower chambers of the heart, called the ventricles.

TETRALOGY OF FALLOT — A congenital malformation of the heart involving four distinct defects (hence tetralogy). Named for Etienne Fallot, French physician who described the condition in 1888. The four defects are:
1. an abnormal opening in the wall between the lower chambers of the heart.
2. misplacement of the aorta, "over-riding" the abnormal opening, so that it receives blood from both the right and left lower chambers instead of only the left.
3. narrowing of the pulmonary artery.
4. enlargement of the right lower chamber of the heart.

THROMBOSIS — The formation or presence of a blood clot (thrombus) inside a blood vessel or cavity of the heart causing a blockage of blood flow.

THROMBUS — A blood clot which forms inside a blood vessel or cavity of the heart.

TRANSPLANTATION — In cancer research, the technique of removing a tumor from one anmial and growing it in the body of another animal of the same species.

TRICUSPID VALVE — A valve consisting of three cusps or triangular segments located between the upper and lower chamber in the right side of the heart. Its position correponds to the bicuspid or mitral valve in the left side of the heart.

TUMOR — An abnormal mass of tissue.

ULTRAVIOLENT — Referring to invisible rays beyond the violet end of the spectrum.

VAGINA — Canal that leads from outer opening of the female reproductive tract to the uterus or womb.

VASOCONSTRICTOR — The vasoconstrictor nerves are one part of the involuntary nervous system. When these nerves are stimulated they cause the muscles of the arterioles to contract, thus narrowing the arteriole passage, increasing the resistance to the flow of blood, and raising the blood pressure. Chemical substances which stimulate the muscles of the arterioles to contract are called vasoconstrictor agents or vasopressors. An example is adrenalin or epinephrine.

VEIN — Any one of a series of vessels of the vascular system which carries blood from various parts of the body back to the heart. All veins in the body conduct unoxygenated blood except the pulmonary veins which conduct freshly oxygenated blood from the lungs back to the heart.

VENTRICLE — One of the two lower chambers of the heart. Left ventricle pumps oxygenated blood through arteries to the body. Right ventricle pumps un-oxygenated blood through pulmonary artery to lungs. Capacity about 85 cc.

X-RAYS — Any radiations of same general nature as light, but of an extremely short wave length.

Index

DATE DUE

RETURNED			
GAYLORD			PRINTED IN U.S.A.